W9-BTO-284

...is Book

valuable tool for parents AND
actical information, backed up
ve been through these problems
have readers keeping this book
within easy reach for use on a regular basis."

— James F. Crowley, MA, President, Community Intervention,
   Inc., Author, *Alliance For Change: A Plan for Community
   Action on Adolescent Drug Abuse*

· · · · ·

"Bravo!! I wish I could hand [this book] out to every parent who brings a
disgruntled, dropping-out kid to counseling. . .and to every therapist I
know who sees teens."

— Barbara Walker, PhD, Counseling Psychologist

· · · · ·

"Nikki Babbit has written a "jewel." I view it as a valuable tool for parents,
school principals and School Board members, school counselors and
teachers, and police officers assigned to schools. It is beautifully written,
and exhibits expertise and a strong sense of compassion and love for the
adolescents and their families who are involved in some stage of
substance abuse."

— Gail A. Allison, MEd, Retired Middle School Principal

· · · · ·

"Dr. Nikki Babbit has provided a calming, thorough step-by-step guide
through the emotional maelstrom of adolescent substance abuse. I have
never seen a book with such useful and poignant quotes to illustrate the
essential points the author is making. This book is a truly valuable
resource for families."

— Barry H. Gordon, PhD, Clinical Psychologist, Author, *Your
   Father, Your Self*

· · · · ·

"Dr. Babbit has captured the struggle, the courage, and the very essence of parents dealing with themselves and their adolescents who are abusing drugs/alcohol."

— Michael E. Matoney, MBA, Adolescent Treatment Program Director

. . . . .

"This book is for all parents of adolescents. While educating in the area of drug and alcohol abuse and how to watch for particular signs, its principles apply to all the struggles parents encounter with teens. This is one book that supports parents rather than pointing fingers at our shortcomings."

— Mother of six children

. . . . .

"This book is an excellent resource for parents with harmfully dependent adolescents. It provides a comprehensive resource, particularly for those who may not know where to turn."

— Mandy Wragg, NCWA, Canadian Youth Counselor

. . . . .

"Dr. Babbit's emphasis on the under-recognition of adolescent substance abuse, and its close relationship to other psychiatric problems including depression, suicide, and aggression, performs a crucial public service. She presents the material in a straightforward, reader-friendly format that should be required reading for parents, teachers, and professionals."

— John Glazer, MD, Director, Division of Child/Adolescent Psychiatry, University of Rochester, NY, School of Medicine

. . . . .

"This book will be very comforting and useful to many parents concerned about the substance use problems of their children. Readers will relate particularly well to the many personal stories and anecdotes the author has gathered to illustrate her points."

— Gloria Chaim, MSW, CSW, Clinical Director, Addiction
Treatment Program for Special Populations, Center for
Addiction and Mental Health, Toronto, Canada

· · · · ·

"This book reached out to me. It would have helped me in the beginning when my family life was collapsing under the weight of my childrens' addiction."

— Mother of two drug addicted teenagers

· · · · ·

"This book provides parents and pastors with support and guidance when confronted with adolescents they suspect may be involved with drugs. I plan to keep several copies on hand and to also make it required reading for our youth counselors."

— Reverend Sharon E. Patch, DMin, Pastor

Adolescent Drug & Alcohol Abuse

*How to Spot It, Stop It,
and Get Help for Your Family*

Adolescent Drug & Alcohol Abuse

How to Spot It, Stop It,
and Get Help for Your Family

Nikki Babbit

O'REILLY®

Beijing • Cambridge • Farnham • Köln • Paris • Sebastopol • Taipei • Tokyo

Adolescent Drug and Alcohol Abuse: How to Spot It, Stop It, and Get Help for Your Family
by Nikki Babbit

Copyright © 2000 O'Reilly & Associates, Inc. All rights reserved. Printed in the United States of America. Published by O'Reilly & Associates, Inc., 101 Morris Street, Sebastopol, CA 95472.

Editor: Linda Lamb

Production Editor: Sarah Jane Shangraw

Cover Design: Kathleen Wilson

Printing History: March 2000: First Edition

Library of Congress Cataloging-in-Publication Data:

Babbit, Nikki, 1941–
    Adolescent drug and alcohol abuse : how to spot it, stop it, and get help for your family
/ Nikki Babbit.—1st ed.
        p. cm.—(Patient-centered guides)
    Includes bibliographical references and index.
    ISBN 1-56592-755-9 (pbk.)
        1. Teenagers—Drug use—Prevention. 2. Teenagers—Alcohol use—Prevention.
    3. Drug abuse—Treatment. 4. Alcoholism—Treatment. 5. Parents of narcotic addicts.
    6. Parents of alcoholics. 7. Parenting. I. Title. II. Series.
HV5824.Y68 B27 2000
649'.4—dc21   99-087517

In memory of my parents, Mary Juno Burch and F. Russell Patch. Their inspirational recoveries taught me that there is always hope for families. Their encouragement taught me that I had the wings to write this book. Their loving spirits were with me on every page.

Table of Contents

Preface

IS MY CHILD INVOLVED with drugs or alcohol? This is a question that haunts most parents of teenagers.

Parents are often the last to know about their children's involvement with alcohol or drugs. I was, even though I knew all the signs and symptoms and had been teaching about them as the director of a treatment program for adolescent drug and alcohol dependency.

On the other hand, I also knew that adolescent drug and alcohol abuse can happen to any teenager, no matter how much drug education he has had, no matter what his socioeconomic level, how much he goes to church, and whether his parents are married or divorced. In addition, substance abuse can happen to any teenager no matter how much her parents know about effective parenting techniques, what neighborhood she lives in, or whether she attends home school, private school, or public school.

I was prepared for the fact that, indeed, my teenager could be an addict/alcoholic. This assessment saved his life.

Adolescent drug and alcohol abusers often do whatever they can to conceal their use. The smarter their parents, the harder they try to cover up what they are doing. Families can rationalize their behaviors, particularly in adolescence, as being caused by something other than drugs or alcohol. Perhaps the defiance is related to an identity crisis. Maybe the challenge to home rules is just part of normal separation from parents. Perhaps the moodiness is due to a breakup with a boyfriend or girlfriend. Maybe all the changes are just the adolescent hormones kicking in.

Our adolescents are living in a drug culture that never existed before. Alcohol continues to be the most easily abused drug because of its availability and the fact that it is socially sanctioned. Binge drinking is on an alarming rise, with the resultant sexual acting out in an unsafe manner, unwanted pregnancies, and deaths of promising young people who had otherwise bright futures.

In addition:

- LSD is now marketed to younger children with colorful designs or cartoon characters.

- Needles are no longer a deterrent to heroin use because heroin is available in a form so pure that it can be snorted.

- Adolescents are stealing drugs from the family medicine cabinet and selling them as party drugs.

- Marijuana and LSD now exist in forms that are more potent than in the 1960s.

- Opium, thought by many parents to exist only in the Far East, is available as a drug of choice for our teenagers.

- Animal tranquilizers and crack or pure cocaine are added to cigarettes or marijuana and smoked at teenage gatherings.

- Underground home laboratories for manufacturing methamphetamine have made this drug much more available for illegal use.

- Dance parties called raves are characterized by the use of drugs such as ecstasy, often added to alcohol without detection until it is too late. Ecstasy can cause severe psychological problems and death. Emergency room admissions involving the drug have risen sharply.

- Common household products are being inhaled by teenagers and can be deadly.

- The average age when teens start drinking alcohol is 13. This means that many are also starting at a younger age.[1]

- The average age when teens start experimenting with marijuana is 14. This means that many are also experimenting at a younger age.[2]

Adolescents think they are invincible. They are aware that there are potential dangers when they use drugs or binge on alcohol, but think they will escape them. They, like adults, minimize their chances of death from inebriation accidents such as drowning in a river, mangling their bodies in a car, or suffocating from vomit.

Why I wrote this book

Facts like these have been part of my professional life for 35 years as I worked with teenagers, first as a high school teacher, then as a school psychologist, then in inner-city mental health agencies and a psychiatric ward, and as the director of an adolescent substance abuse agency where I also facilitated family therapy groups and parent education/support groups for close to 20 years. I had firsthand knowledge of the struggles parents have in getting help for their teenagers, a struggle I appreciated even more when one of my own children went to treatment at age 17. I realized how parents blame themselves when this happens, how issues from their own childhood affect their parenting in this painful situation, how even good marriages like mine are severely tested, and how parents have to deal with the frustration of not being able to make their teenagers well.

As the daughter and stepdaughter of alcoholics, I had hoped that through good parenting and the power of example that my own children would escape substance abuse. I knew intellectually that addiction or alcoholism can happen to anyone, but deep down, on an emotional level, I thought I could prevent it in my own family. My teenager's treatment taught me a profound lesson on the emotional level that made me a better parent and enriched my work with alcoholics and addicts. The experience also deepened my commitment to spread knowledge, strength, and hope to others. I became more active in teaching and consulting all over the United States and even had the opportunity to help bring Alcoholics Anonymous (AA), Al-Anon (a self-help support group for family members of alcoholics/addicts), and western treatment methods to Russia.

This book gave me the opportunity to tell the story of what parents go through when they suspect their adolescents might be abusing drugs or alcohol. I have worked with thousands of parents and know that the books available do not often provide the voices of those who have been there. I wanted to integrate information that parents are looking for with personal accounts of their struggles. This would be an additional way to spread knowledge, strength, and hope.

What this book offers

This book helps all parents of pre-teenagers and teenagers whether or not they suspect that their young people are using drugs and alcohol. For those who are not struggling, it illuminates what could lie ahead and gives information ahead of time that may help to stave off delays when action is needed. For parents who do suspect abuse or dependency, this book gives information, support, and guidance.

This book can also be helpful to grandparents, aunts and uncles, and friends of parents of pre-teenagers and teenagers. These parents need support, and the book shows how to support them.

In addition, this book will be helpful to pediatricians, child and adolescent psychiatrists and psychologists, therapists, teachers, school administrators and guidance counselors, church youth workers and pastors, probation officers, judges, referees, and elected officials who want to hear the voices of parents struggling with their teenagers' substance abuse, addiction, or alcoholism, and where to get help for their teens and themselves. These voices illustrate the pain and frustration of trying to help your adolescent children while being judged by society. The voices of the parents tell a story of what is happening in our culture, but is rarely talked about.

Language in the book

Even though alcohol is a drug, I have used the word alcohol next to drugs as if they are different. The general culture puts less attention on alcohol as a problem than drugs, partly because it is legal and it is more socially acceptable. This is dangerous thinking because alcohol-related accidents and deaths are greater than any other mood-altering substance. I wanted to call attention to alcohol being of equal concern.

Secondly, I used the words teenagers or adolescents to mean young people of both genders rather than alternating the singular pronouns he and she. It is also my experience that parents sometimes have several adolescents who are drug/alcohol abusers or alcoholics/addicts.

How this book is organized

I have organized this book to parallel most parents' experiences as they live with, and get help for, their drug/alcohol-abusing adolescents. Many of the chapters overlap because everything is happening at the same time. For example, parents need to understand what is going on with drug/alcohol abuse (Chapter 1) at the same time that they seek an assessment (Chapter 3), at the same time that they examine their own feelings (Chapter 5) and their relationships and communication (Chapter 7), at the same time that they start to work on their own recovery (Chapter 8), and when letting go (Chapter 9). Chapter 10 helps parents with how to provide natural consequences for their teenagers. It is best to first skim the entire book to see everything it contains. Then you will have an overview of your journey. Once that is accomplished, you can use each chapter as a more detailed guide for your follow-up action.

From working with overwhelmed parents for many years, and from having those periods when I, too, was overwhelmed, I know that reading a book is difficult when you are emotionally spent and burnt out. Therefore, I have tried to keep the chapters "reader friendly" by eliminating technical jargon and imposing studies.

The words of parents and professionals who work with parents are set off in italics. Their experience is offered to give reassurance that no matter what is happening to those who are reading, they are not the only ones who have ever felt that way or engaged in the same behaviors. Quite the contrary. Although I interviewed more than 30 parents in person for the book, their voices mirror the thousands of parents I have worked with who have struggled with their teenagers' drug abuse and dependency. These were voices of parents from as dissimilar locations as Sanibel Island, Florida, and Toronto, Canada; Houston, Texas, and Moscow, Russia; Cleveland, Ohio, and Helsinki, Finland. Parents all over the world, despite differences in language, are united in their common concern about drug/alcohol abuse and dependency in their children. They share the common fear of losing their children because of this abuse and dependency, and they attend support groups such as Nar-Anon, Families Anonymous, or Al-Anon, which are in more than 130 countries around the world.

The parents who directly participated in the book did so with a desire to help others like themselves. These parents can become a support system for those who are turning to this book for ideas and empowerment. Words from young people who struggled with drug/alcohol abuse and addiction are also included. They are healthier now, and their stories will help parents better understand what is going on with their own adolescents. Addicts/alcoholics who have been in recovery for at least fifteen years also share their insights, experiences, and encouragement.

I have included a "Taking care of yourself" section at the end of each chapter with suggestions for supportive activities and reading. Appendix A gives many more suggestions. Appendix B gives information on support groups, drug prevention and treatment, parent mobilization groups, and parenting web sites. Appendix C gives detailed information on drugs that are currently being used by teenagers.

What you will find in this book is a wealth of information and practical, personal advice from parents who have experienced what it is like to have drug/alcohol-abusing adolescents. One cannot help but admire them for their struggle. The last chapter, *Stories of Empowerment*, shows their triumph and the fact that if teenagers do not decide to get well, their parents can. This is a book of encouragement, and of hope for the future.

Acknowledgements

I have been deeply grateful in my life to be inspired, encouraged, and supported by so many wonderful people. This book is filled with a basketful of their blessings.

First of all, I wish to thank Jim Crowley of Community Intervention, Minneapolis, Minnesota, who asked me to write a booklet in 1988 about substance abuse following the experience with my own teenager. His support at that time, and for this expanded project, has been central to my motivation as well as encouragement to our family to share our story in order to help others.

I would also like to thank four widely published nonfiction writers—Peggy Anderson, Hope Edelman, Michel Marriott, and Musa Mayer—who encouraged me in the last twelve years to expand the booklet. I studied under them at summer writers' workshops at Antioch College and the University of Iowa. They honed my skills in nonfiction writing and energized me to continue to grow.

Central to the completion of this project is also Jean Lewis, whom I met at one of my many Antioch workshops. We have encouraged each other in our writing, and I have learned how important it is for writers to have cheerleaders in their lives.

Two other significant cheerleaders for this book were my friend Karen Burt and my editor at O'Reilly, Linda Lamb. I have titled Karen "Queen of the Most Patient and Reassuring." She was able to go beyond the hopelessness of my eighth-grade typing teacher who failed me twice, but made a deal with the principal that she would stay in her job if I could be made exempt from the school requirement. I was determined to learn how to use my computer and word processor to type this entire book. Karen taught me how to do it. Central School in Glencoe, Illinois, can be proud that I finally passed. I feel accomplished that I can now keep up with the computing skills of my three-year-old grandson, Brandon Babbit, and others his age, who will move quickly ahead of me. Such is the challenge for the older generation in this computer age!

Linda Lamb is every writer's dream of an editor. Not only is she talented, intelligent, and perceptive, she reads all of your work in a timely manner and with a careful eye and encourages you to keep going. I have had so many writer friends tell me how fortunate I am to have her support. "I know," I tell them. "I know." Linda's name appeared many times in my gratitude journal while I was writing this book.

I am especially grateful to those talented, perceptive individuals in the United States and Canada who agreed to read the manuscript for this project before the final printing. They were consultants with schools or courts, school professionals, adolescent and family therapists, adolescent addiction/alcoholism treatment professionals, clergy, or parents. Their associations with the material represented those who would read the book once it was published. I had much more confidence about the final product after integrating their suggestions for improvement. Their support and encouragement nourished me and was invaluable. In alphabetical order, they are: Gail Allison, MEd; Gloria Chaim, MSW, CSW; Jim Crowley, MA; John Glazer, MD; Barry Gordon, PhD; Cathy Hugney, RN; Mike and Sheri Lohuis; Mike Matoney, MBA; Rev. Sharon E. Patch, DMin; Barbara Walker, PhD; and Mandy Wragg, NCWA.

I am also deeply grateful to the talented staff in the Patient-Centered Guides division of O'Reilly & Associates who were so helpful: Shawnde Paull for coordinating the book through production with enthusiasm and skill, Carol Wenmoth for dedicating her keen eye to a helpful edit, and Lisa Olson for her creative talents. One of the most fascinating aspects of this project has been learning how a book goes from the first sentence on an author's page to sitting on the shelf in a library or bookstore.

I have special thanks for those who helped create this book by agreeing to be interviewed; sharing ideas, assistance, or material; or offering continued encouragement and enthusiastic, witty notes to keep me going. Their names are also listed alphabetically: Laurie Artz, Jan Balmat, Helen Bassett, Jan Bennet, Agnes Boehnlein, Elder Oliver D. Bouie, Craig Cunningham, Rev. Jim Dowd, Debbie F., Gary F., Mike F., Gary Gottlieb, MD, Melissa Guerrero,

Nancy Gustafson, Velma Hughes, Jim Joyner, Ann Kent, Rachel Kugelman, Rev. Laury Larson, Carol M., Francine McNulty, Lennie Meades, Roxie Michener, John Naccarato, Keila Naparstek, Sally Newman, Carl Pastard, Donnie Pastard, Occie Pastard, Dianne Pexa, Jim Pexa, Juliane Schnell, Sandy Slessinger, John Thomas, Liz Timko, Aloen Townsend, John Wagner, Jeff Ward, Debbie Wasson, Doug Wasson, Dennis Wert, Vicki Wert, Karyn West, Vickie, and Larry. Others are not listed because they wish to remain anonymous.

Finally, I wish to express profound gratitude for my husband of 35 years, Harold Babbit, and my children, Ross, Jamie, and Rider. They have supported my writing and my professional commitments over many years in so many ways. Harold, in particular, has encouraged my relentless focus that can sometimes be tiring to others, and his serenity on this project was my continual anchor. His humor, his fish dinners, and his flowers were the flame that kept my light burning.

Thanks to all of those named and unnamed for being in my life. You have surrounded me with your circle of love, and I am profoundly changed as a result. This book, and the writing of it, with all the people I have met and been inspired by, has deepened me more than I would have ever thought possible. What wonderful gifts to take with me as I begin a new century.

—Nikki Babbit
Shaker Heights (Cleveland), Ohio
January 2000

If you would like to comment on this book or offer suggestion for future editions, send email to *patientguides@oreilly.com*, or write to O'Reilly & Associates, Inc. at 101 Morris Street, Sebastopol, CA 95472.

CHAPTER 1

Use, Abuse, and Dependency

When the most important things in our life
happen, we quite often do not know at the
moment what is going on.

—C. S. Lewis

IS YOUR TEENAGER ABUSING drugs or alcohol? Parents are often the last to know. This is because those who have developed a harmful relationship with drugs and alcohol cover it up, even to themselves, in order to continue. Parents often attribute their teenager's misbehavior to other causes or think that because they have strong family values or live in the right community, their teenager could not possibly have drug problems.

This chapter will explore common misconceptions about the chances of alcohol and drug abuse being a problem in a family. We will then discuss how drug or alcohol abuse affects the abuser, and what is happening at the same time to the user's family. Drug and alcohol abuse often leads to confusion, denial, and excuses within the family. As a result, abusers may not get the help they need.

Common misconceptions

As children grow, parents watch them deal with such problems as rejection on the playground, not getting a star on a spelling test (despite practicing from their mother's dictation the night before), not being chosen for a sports team, or hearing about someone they know being killed in a traffic accident. Parents weather these disappointments with their children and try to offer their support. As children grow up, they may have to cope with other disturbing events, such as breaking up with a girlfriend or boyfriend; having to deal with death or divorce; having a parent lose their job; the family farm being sold to developers; having to adjust to a new school, a new neighborhood, or even a move across the country.

Parents know that events like these have an impact on children and adolescents. It is easy to think that "acting out" behaviors are a result of these events. Parents can feel sorry for young people who have gone through these struggles, and these feelings can help to justify their misbehavior, no matter how destructive. Parents may use such excuses for months or even years after the original event.

Parents might easily overlook their teenager's drug abuse because they attribute the related misbehavior to another event. These events, and teens' observable reactions to them, may disguise substance abuse behavior. Parents of drug-addicted teens who did not know their children were on drugs describe what they thought was really going on:

> I had to be gone a lot in my job, but I was really a devoted father when I was home. When our son started misbehaving, I felt guilty about my absences. I thought that this was why he was having so much trouble.

· · · · ·

> My husband and I went through a painful divorce a few years before and I just thought my daughter was struggling with that.

· · · · ·

> The transition to high school involved a bigger school, so my wife and I thought that this was why our son got into so much trouble.

· · · · ·

> My son broke up with his really nice girlfriend, so my husband and I thought that if they got back together everything would clear up with all his misbehavior.

· · · · ·

> My daughter was always on the sensitive side, so when she had mood swings in high school, my wife and I thought that she was just too sensitive. She couldn't handle things that happen to normal kids. [We thought this was] why she was having so many problems.

Unfortunately, these parents did not realize that drug abuse could be going on, and no one encouraged them to at least rule out drugs and alcohol as a cause of their adolescent's misbehavior. The mother of a drug-addicted and now drug-free teen explains her regrets:

> *I wish that someone had encouraged us to get an assessment in an earlier stage. The behaviors were all there. But it was easier to think of another cause than to check it out by going to someone to do an evaluation. And since we didn't go earlier, my son just got deeper and deeper into his drugs. We almost lost him once in a bad LSD trip. He just freaked out. It was scary. I've heard about kids who never come back from that, and then they jump off bridges and kill themselves. We were lucky that we got help before that happened.*

When adolescents start hanging around people their parents don't approve of or start doing things that result in legal trouble, it is easy to attribute these behaviors to normal adolescent rebellion. It is also easy to blame problems on new friends, peer pressure, or the wrong choices. Even when parents question the role that drugs might play, it is easy to dismiss it, particularly when the child denies there is a problem. One father relates his story:

> *Our son was well on his way in his addiction, but when we questioned him about drugs maybe being a problem he was pretty angry. He said something like, "Do you really think I'd be that stupid?" We wanted to believe that his behavior was related to all the moves we had, and we had really taught him well about the dangers of drugs, so we believed him.*

This father's story illustrates another misconception: if you teach your children well, they will not have problems with drugs. Parents and school personnel can overlook drug or alcohol abuse when they have a strong anti-drug education program in their home or school. The assumption is that this education will prevent abuse. That sounds logical, but it doesn't always work for all kids.

The mother of an alcoholic teen explains how she tried to educate her children about alcoholism:

> *Both of my own parents had a lot of problems with alcoholism. They were even out of control when we had family visits with them. We talked about it at home with the idea that our kids would never choose this kind of life for themselves. We were sure that our kids got the point. I mean, how could they miss it?*

A recovering alcoholic mother describes a similar misconception that results in blinders about drug and alcohol abuse:

> When my two daughters were growing up, I was in recovery. I even took them to AA meetings with me. I really beat myself up when I didn't see that they had the same symptoms that were part of my own alcoholism. I blamed these behaviors on other things. Since my girls saw how much happier I was without drinking, I thought that they would feel the same way. They certainly wouldn't choose the life of an alcoholic.

All of these misconceptions about the causes of alcoholism and addiction assume that potential addicts or alcoholics are capable of making decisions to control their substance use, and that they know the right thing to do. A teen addict/alcoholic who is now attending Alcoholics Anonymous (AA) meetings in order to remain sober and drug-free describes his blinders:

> I knew that my grandparents lost most of their lives because of alcoholism. I also lived in a loving home where my parents didn't have alcohol in the house, and we talked about the dangers of addiction. So I thought that I would never be an addict. And I would make sure that if I drank, it would never get out of control. No way! I was too smart to let that happen.

Many writers, such as Claudia Black in her book, *It Will Never Happen to Me*, have explored the myth that knowledge allows a person to escape addiction. Black is an assessment professional who has diagnosed hundreds of adult and adolescent addicts. She explains:

> Knowledge can lead to a false sense of security where addiction is concerned. Family members of addicts are sure that it will never happen to them because they want to avoid inflicting the same pain on others. Parents think that because their child has been raised under the right circumstances, they will escape. The fact of the matter is, it can happen to anyone. Even when we think that it should happen to someone who had parents who were drunk around the kids or who lived with addicts next door, they escape. The disease is unpredictable. It provides equal opportunity to everyone.

Use, abuse, and dependency

Anyone, therefore, can become an alcoholic and addict, but many will also escape. As Vernon Johnson, DD, a world-recognized authority on alcoholism and addiction who died in 1999, explains:

> It's clear that all sorts of people become drug and alcohol dependent, some for no apparent reason. On the other hand, it seems that some people can't become dependent no matter how hard they try!

> We do know that drug and alcohol dependence isn't caused by a lack of will power, weakness of character, or some flaw in a person's moral structure. And it's not a form of mental illness. Nor is it the result of external influences—an unhappy marriage, trouble on the job, peer pressure.[1]

Johnson reminds us that there is no absolute reason that explains the cause of addiction. There is a simple truth: no matter what parents have done, they did not cause their adolescent's drug abuse or addiction.

> This means that if someone you care about is alcoholic or dependent on other drugs, it's not your fault. You're not responsible for the disease of dependence that has taken hold in the person that you care about. You may be feeling guilty anyway; but try to believe—or at least consider— that nothing you've ever done could have caused that person's illness.[2]

Parents may feel skeptical about not blaming themselves because they have heard parents blamed for children's problems in the newspaper or from relatives. These judgmental comments are not accurate when they are applied to alcoholism or addiction. The disease model that follows is a more accurate explanation than looking for blame.

The biopsychosocial disease model

How do abuse and dependency happen? The biopsychosocial disease model defines the disease of addiction as primary, progressive, chronic, and ultimately fatal if not arrested. The disease is characterized by the ongoing use of drugs or alcohol despite harmful consequences. It is also described as a no-fault illness, like diabetes, because alcoholics and addicts do not *choose* to be dependent. According to this model, treatment needs to address the biological, psychological, and social aspects of the disease.

This disease model is widely accepted by both physicians and professional groups all over the United States and Canada, and the model is emulated in many other areas of the world. In the 1980s, Mikhail Gorbachev instructed government officials in the Soviet Union to go to the United States to study this disease model so it could be used to address the serious alcoholism problem that was undermining Soviet society. Treatment professionals from the United States and members of AA and Al-Anon, a family support program, were then invited to the Soviet Union to help begin this new approach to treating alcoholics. Up until that time, treatment in the Soviet Union consisted of making alcoholics violently ill by giving them alcohol along with anti-alcohol medication. AA had not been allowed because public meetings were forbidden. Also, it was stated that alcoholism only occurred in capitalist countries. An adolescent treatment professional who made two trips to Russia at that time describes the significance of what was happening:

> I really appreciated how lucky we are to treat alcoholics with compassion and according to the disease model when I saw how desperately the Soviet medical profession was trying to learn how to do this.

The biopsychosocial disease model is used as the model for treatment by the American Medical Association, the American Psychiatric Association, the American Hospital Association, the American Public Health Association, the American Psychological Association, the National Association of Social Workers, the World Health Organization, and the American College of Physicians.[3] It is also used as a model for treatment by the Joint Commission on Accreditation for Healthcare Organizations (JCAHO), by insurance plans in the United States that will help parents pay for their children's treatment, and by many provinces in Canada. In both the United States and Canada, certain aspects of the model may be emphasized more than others in treatment, and spiritual degeneration may also be addressed. The model may have a different emphasis in some Canadian provinces. A Canadian treatment professional from Vancouver explains:

> Although the biopsychosocial model can and does include the disease concept in its biological component, some of us in Canada are hesitant to agree with the word disease as part of the model. The biopsychosocial model speaks to matching the approach most suited to client's needs and level of substance involvement whether it is misuse or dependence.

A treatment professional in Toronto adds another aspect of some differences with the United States:

> *Many of the treatment professionals in Canada tend to work more with the harm reduction model, which is not really a phrase you hear as much in the United States. On the other hand, there are also others who treat based on the usual pattern in the United States, which talks about abstinence, using the Twelve Step Program, etc. It varies across the country.*

More information about disease model treatment using the Twelve Step approach will be discussed in Chapter 4, *Treatment/Rehabilitation*. Resources on the harm reduction model can be found in Appendix A, *Resources*.

The biological nature of addiction in particular is also an active area of research in hopes that some day there will be an effective way for addicts and alcoholics to use medication as one of the tools for recovery. Enoch Gordis, MD, director of the National Institute on Alcohol Abuse and Alcoholism, who presented current research at an August 1999 international meeting on alcoholism, states:

> *With the neuroscience cooking along as it is, and the prospect that we'll find genes related to alcoholism, we would have far more targeted drug therapies for alcoholism in the next five to ten years.*[4]

A 1997 *Time* magazine article entitled "How We Get Addicted" discussed the generally accepted theory that addiction occurs because alcohol and drugs act on several important neurotransmitters and their receptors on brain cells, with both acute and long-term effects. Much of the research focuses on the elevation of a brain chemical called dopamine. Certain individuals, for reasons that are not totally understood, are more susceptible to this elevation than others. Even inherited genetic factors are no guarantee that you will or will not experience this effect.[5] The simple fact is, one person will get hooked, another will not.

Stages in the progression of the disease

Although we still have much to learn about the causes of alcoholism and addiction, we do know a great deal about the progression from drugs use and alcohol to abuse to eventual dependency. We know how this happens, why it happens, and how this progression is harmful to abusers and their families. It is helpful to understand this process so as to be able to intervene sooner to prevent serious harm and, if one is a chronic addict/alcoholic, death.

Stage one: Learning about mood-altering substances

The social use of alcohol is commonly accepted in our culture. In addition, many of us learned from our first experiences with alcohol that even one glass of wine or beer affects the way we feel, usually in a pleasant way. We learned, as promised in the many ads we see on television or on billboards that we relaxed, lightened up, and enjoyed ourselves when we had a drink or two. We learned that the upward swing in our mood happened every time we drank, and that the degree of the swing increased the more we drank. In short, we learned the pleasurable effects of alcohol.

We also learned what happens when we drink more than we can handle. Our mood still continues in an upward swing, but, past a certain point, there are some unpleasant consequences as well. Those drinking too much might be embarrassed, for example, because their loud and talkative behavior or flushed cheeks reveal that they have had too much to drink. Others may become combative or even abusive when under the influence of alcohol or drugs. Some might feel sick the next day.

Stage two: Seeking the mood swing

The discovery of the unpleasant effects of alcohol represents an important turning point that influences whether or not a person will go on to substance abuse. At this point, the negative effects are still reversible. The drinker can recover from one experience with embarrassment or a hangover, and next time, foregoes the greater upswing in mood in order to avoid the subsequent discomfort.

On the other hand, some drinkers decide the maximum high is worth whatever pain they experience as a result of exceeding their limit. They can also decide that the negative consequences can be rationalized away.

Two teens describe their different perceptions of the consequences of drinking:

> I get very light-headed when I drink, and I can feel it after just one beer. I don't like the feeling, and it keeps me from having a good time. So I stop with just one.

• • • • •

*I learned early that I can't tolerate alcohol, but I didn't care. The
high was worth it. And when I kept drinking more, and did really stupid
things, I rationalized that I had had a bad day at school or my parents
were on my back too much. It didn't really matter that I had consequences. I liked using, and I wanted to continue with it no matter what
anyone said. If negative things happened as a result, I just blamed outside forces for how I was acting.*

Humans of any age can go through the denial, delusion, and rationalization
process when seeking a mood swing with drugs or alcohol. Some, like the
first teen, do not—they recognize unpleasant consequences as a signal that
exceeding their limit is not in their best interest. Others, similar to the second teen, an alcoholic, focus on what drinking does *for* them and minimize
the reality of what it does *to* them. Notice by what the alcoholic teen said
that there is often a blaming of someone or something, such as parents or a
bad day, to further justify the drinking behavior. There is also an element of
self-pity that feeds the rationalization.

Teen addicts who entered treatment and are now sober show further how
chemical abusers and addicts think:

*My mom was on my case all the time, so I needed to get high with
my friends just to get away from her. Of course I didn't want to admit to
myself that she had a right to be on my case because of all the trouble I
was in. I persuaded myself that I deserved to get high because she was
such a witch.*

• • • • •

*My parents were on my case all the time because I got in trouble once
for showing up high at school. I kept doing it, but I just got better at hiding it. I rationalized that school was stupid, so it didn't matter if I was
high when I got there.*

• • • • •

*I was mad at my parents for sending me to a therapist so I thought it
was fine that I lied to him about my drug use. Actually, I thought that my
therapist was so stupid he couldn't tell the difference between a lie and the
truth. That's what I focused on when I went to therapy. It was a joke to
me.*

My friends and I thought that everyone in our community was too uptight, so it didn't matter that we did the vandalism we did. Anyway, we were high when we did it, and we just thought it was another good time.

As these addicts and alcoholics illustrate, denial, delusion, and rationalization, accompanied by self-pity, constitute the engine that moves the substance abuse and addiction process forward. In addition, those who are abusing drugs and alcohol have the sincere belief that their problems will go away if they can change other people, something they are doing, or something in their environment. This sincere belief, their self-delusion, traps them in their harmful progression. As this former teen addict explains, delusion goes with blindness:

As I look back, I went to treatment totally convinced that I would show the treatment staff and my parents that I was not an addict. And I was really mad at my parents that they were taking me to this hospital to get help for something that wasn't even a problem. This was really hard for my parents because I had put them through hell. But I was so deluded, and I had an excuse for everything that I was doing. When I started to work on my addiction, of course I saw how blind I really was. I look back now and see how powerful the disease really is. But the practicing addict can't see it.

Stage three: Harmful abuse, harmful dependency

Those adolescents who keep abusing drugs and alcohol despite harmful consequences move further and further along the continuum of abuse to dependency. Even when they are sober, they are in pain. Their environment may be chaotic; they may not feel well physically; others may be angry with them; they may be racked with shame or sadness. They no longer use mood-altering chemicals to feel better than normal—they never even feel as good as normal used to feel. Now they are using to blot out the pain of their consequences. They keep using because their earlier experiences taught them that using drugs and alcohol made them feel good. Using used to work every time to elevate their mood.

During this stage of moving from harmful abuse to dependency, however, the emotional price for using mood-altering chemicals becomes greater. There is the delusion for addicts that they are moving in a positive direction.

In fact, the consequences from using send them deeper into emotional—and often physical—pain.

A teen addict who is now sober relates how emotional pain worsens:

> *As I look back, the simple solution to all my problems was just to use more often. I thought that I would feel better if I could just get more drugs. What a delusion. My progression got worse and worse and I had even more emotional pain as a result.*

A treatment professional who has worked with adults and adolescents explains how deterioration and harmful abuse go together:

> *When addicts enter treatment, they are deteriorating in all areas of their lives: socially, physically, emotionally, intellectually, and spiritually. Drugs and alcohol are being used to relieve guilt, fear, and anxiety about their consequences. They are more and more preoccupied with using drugs and alcohol to cover up these feelings. The pain goes deeper and deeper. There is the vicious cycle of using to cover up the pain, but then having to use because of it.*

Stage four: Chronic and fatal addiction

If addicts do not receive help for their addiction early on, it will progress to chronic dependency. Still deluded that drugs or alcohol will work *for* them, they use because they are in such pain, but in fact, they never move much beyond that low point. Their lives are falling apart, and deep within their psyche, they know it.

Blackouts are longer and more frequent, and there are many physical problems because addicts will often ignore their nutritional needs and their resistance to infection is low. There is a desperation to get high, often to prevent the pain of withdrawal. Suspicious thinking increases because of memory loss due to blackouts. At this stage, addicts/alcoholics usually have high anxiety about their behaviors and increased guilt. They feel helpless and hopeless. But, as an adult addict with many years of sobriety relates, they still want to keep using drugs and alcohol:

> *When I went from being a graduate of Notre Dame with a highly successful career in radio to an alcoholic bum on the streets, I still believed that if only I could get another drink, my troubles would all go away.*

This is the power of alcoholism and addiction. Addicts at this stage are very depressed and still undertake an often-futile search for another drink or drug to take the pain away. They may also decide that the best way to end their pain is to end their lives. Another adult who has been sober for years explains how pain can lead to death:

> Before I went to treatment the last time, I tried to hang myself in a cell when I was picked up for a DUI. I knew that my life was at a really low point, and I didn't think that there was any hope for me. When I read stories in the paper about people who succeed with suicide, I really feel sad. If only they could have gotten help like I did.

Evidence of the despair of chronic addicts is all around us if we look. Some citizens of Portland, Oregon, were reminded of the desperation in the chronic stage when they were driving home from work on July 1, 1998, and saw two bodies hanging from a steel bridge, twin nooses slipped around their necks. The couple in their 20s, Michael Douglas and fiancée Mora McGowan, were heroin addicts whose habit left them with unmanageable lives and no hope. Douglas left a journal that described their decision to end their lives.

The 1998 *Time* magazine article entitled "Public Suicide Awakens City to Problem of Drug Addiction" describes this event, focusing the couple's despair:

> Those who knew Douglas said that drugs were always part of his life. When he and McGowan began using heroin, they started pawning every-thing they owned of any value to feed their habit. They were eventually kicked out of the friend's apartment where they had been staying and put on the streets.

> At least once, McGowan tried treatment but failed. In despair, she tried suicide by cutting her wrists, but her mother rushed her to a hospi-tal. Douglas tried to come up with the money to buy enough heroin for an overdose, but he couldn't.

> Police Sgt. Kent Perry said Douglas wrote in his journal about the grind of having to raise $200 every day to pay for his fix and how he con-sidered other ways of ending his life, including shooting himself or lying down on train tracks.[6]

This story shows how much despair exists in chronic addicts. It also summarizes the disease model of addiction and illustrates the co-existence of drug dependency and other psychiatric disorders such as depression and suicidal thinking. Drug dependency was primary, progressive, chronic, and fatal in those young persons' lives.

Substance abuse can progress to dependency if it is not stopped. The illness can become chronic and end with addicts taking their own lives. Fatalities can also occur from acts of poor judgment such as accidental overdoses and automobile and boating accidents. The daily newspaper is filled with stories of such needless deaths.

Stages in family progression

While potential drug and alcohol abusers are learning about the effects of drugs and alcohol, and perhaps progressing from use to abuse to dependency, their families also go through predictable stages.

Stage one: Attempts to adjust

Based on the fact that alcohol is an acceptable mood-altering chemical in our society, families often accept someone in the family being high or drunk as normal, even when their behaviors are confusing, embarrassing, and painful. If an adolescent's use continues at this stage, parents usually appeal to their logic in hopes that they will be smart and stop what they are doing. They tell their teens that driving while drunk would not be safe, acting foolish at a family gathering would be disrespectful, people can get fired if they show up drunk at work or be suspended if they are drunk at school. Parents may impose restrictions or a new curfew if the consequences of drinking get out of hand.

In attempts to adjust, family members often start to rescue drug and alcohol abusers by doing chores for them or waking them up when they used to need only their alarm clock. It is common for parents at this stage to feel vulnerable and to start blaming their children's friends, their school, their community, the other parent, or even in-laws for all the problems. Parents may even resort to spending money on a new school, moving, or taking other actions to try to control a situation that is becoming out of control. Chapter 5, *Working on Your Feelings*, and Chapter 6, *Harmful Consequences from Normal Feelings*, elaborate on common feelings and actions of parents.

Loved ones may also rescue chemical abusers by getting them out of jail. One father of an addict relates how he ended up paying a heavy price for this behavior:

> We didn't like the idea of our daughter staying overnight in jail, so we posted ten percent of the bond. Our daughter came home, and then she ran away. She was still on the run when we had the court hearing, and we had to come up with the full $10,000. We also got a lecture from a judge who told us that the trouble with society these days is that parents can't take care of their kids. That was a little hard to take since what we had done was to try and take care of her, and now we were out $10,000.

At this stage of adjustment, it is normal to suspect that drug/alcohol use might be a problem. On the other hand, it is easy to see using as a symptom of some other problem and to seek counseling help. Well-trained therapists know to consider substance abuse in any teenager coming to them for any problem. Many adolescents will not admit their drug/alcohol use, however, and will blame their problems on their parents, school, friends, or whatever else is part of their own denial system. Unfortunately, untrained therapists can make unhealthy alliances with substance abusers and start to blame the parents as well. The key fact, however, is that family members are already in their own denial, and they join the substance abuser, and even the therapist, in what can best be described as a denial dance. Two parents of addicts relate how denial affected them:

> The therapist our son was seeing told us he didn't have a drug problem. That's what we wanted to believe, so we accepted it. On the other hand, he said that we needed to give our son more freedom and that was the real problem. We were confused because he was going out at night and doing other things that we thought needed consequences. But we felt we had to trust the therapist, so that's what we did. We found out later that our son lied to the therapist about his drug use and talked the therapist into thinking that all the problems were our fault. We were upset that the therapist had handled it so poorly, but we were willing to believe that our son wasn't the problem, we were.

· · · · ·

> I grew up in an alcoholic home and, as a result, it was easy for me as a mother to be in denial and to not trust my instincts. When my daughter

got in trouble, I suspected drugs as a cause, but when a therapist who wasn't trained in addiction didn't see it, I was too afraid to speak up. My instincts were correct, but I dismissed them.

These parents show the pain, frustration, and denial that are part of the adjustment stage. Unfortunately, however, if alcoholics and addicts are progressing in their use, this denial can be catastrophic. A mother who has lived for years with the consequences of her son's LSD use explains:

Our son was very secretive about his use in the earlier stages, but at least we took him to a therapist because we knew that something was wrong. He told his therapist that we were too strict. We needed to loosen up. We know now that he really manipulated the therapist, but at the time we went along with this and gave our son more freedom. One night he went out with friends and had a really bad trip on LSD. He hasn't been the same since, and it has been years.

This story also illustrates that in the adjustment stage, drug and alcohol abusers can often become the center of attention; families adjust their roles or behaviors to accommodate them.

Stage two: Isolation

When families have adolescent substance abusers and family members have accommodated to them in a dance of denial, it is normal for parents to become isolated. One mother of an addict explains how this isolation worked:

We were too afraid to leave the house for fear of what our son would do while we were gone, so we stopped going out. And we were too afraid that he might start a big fight or something, so we stopped inviting people over. We made a lot of excuses about being busy. Our friends thought we were just too busy for them, and that we were dropping hints that we no longer wanted them as friends. The fact of the matter was that we were desperate for friends, but we were too afraid to tell people what was going on.

This mother illustrates another characteristic of the isolation stage: the fear of talking about family problems with outsiders. There is silence inside the family as well. Alcoholism and drug dependency are often described as elephants in the living room that no one admits they notice. Denial of this elephant is easy because it goes hand in hand with fear, emotional and physical pain, and blaming oneself for what is going on. Isolation keeps this pattern going. When isolation occurs, it is impossible for a family or a substance abuser to get help.

Stage three: Unhealthy surrender to the illness

If the stages progress without intervention from outsiders who correctly perceive that there is substance abuse going on in the home, it is easy for families to give up trying to do anything about the problems that are tearing them apart. It is common for individual family members to overcompensate by being extra good, whereas others may act out and become the center of attention. It is easy to feel that something is wrong with the family and to isolate even further as a result.

As this stage moves along, drug and alcohol abusers have progressed in their own disease, so their behaviors may now include running away. There is a mixed blessing to this, as one mother of an addict explains:

> My husband and I felt guilty that we were relieved when our son didn't come home for two weeks. But at least we had a break from all the fights, and we could pay attention to our daughters. We were tired of everything that was happening, but we had also given up. It was just too much effort to fight anymore. We let our son do whatever he wanted. Fights over consequences were just too draining. We stopped giving consequences, too.

During this stage, family members often experience stress-related illnesses. A mother describes how this happened to her:

> When I was growing up in an alcoholic home, I got sick a lot from losing sleep at night or worrying. When our daughter was having all her problems with drugs, I went back to the same types of illnesses where I had to call in sick to work.

This mother illustrates that patterns in this stage can revert back to how problems were handled as a child.

Lastly, an even greater consequence of progression to the stress in this last stage is that marriages can suffer and parents may decide that the only solution to their problems is to get a divorce. The mother of an addict who has been sober for almost fifteen years explains how drug use affected her marriage:

My husband and I blamed each other for everything that was happening with our daughter. When marriage counseling didn't seem to be working, we both thought that we would have to get a divorce. We were not thinking that the real problem was that our daughter was an addict. The therapist we were seeing didn't even raise that possibility even though how we were acting was typical of the split that couples often have.

I was angry for a while that the therapist didn't raise the possibility of drug abuse, but then someone told me that therapists aren't always trained for this. Thank God we got to some professionals who figured out the truth. We didn't get a divorce, and we are about to celebrate our 35th anniversary. We're more in love than ever.

Taking care of yourself

It is important to prevent isolation and hopelessness. These can be overcome by specific actions. These actions will lead to increased knowledge and empowerment.

Find a support meeting

As parents struggle with whether or not there is alcohol and drug abuse in their family, it is normal to feel confused and isolated. Therefore, one of the first steps to empowerment is to seek out support from others. Families Anonymous and Al-Anon exist to help parents with this support. Nar-Anon, similar to Al-Anon and specifically for family members of narcotic abusers, has many meetings in Canada, although there are fewer in the United States. It will be important to find a meeting online or in your community and to begin attending immediately.

Al-Anon groups began in the 1940s. They are in communities all over the United States and Canada, online, and in more than 80 countries around the world. Families Anonymous groups started in the 1970s, and they are in many communities as well.

Who goes to these Twelve Step groups? Anyone who is affected by someone's drinking or drug use can attend. Al-Anon was begun by Lois Wilson, the wife of one of the founders of Alcoholics Anonymous. She and several of her friends realized that their own lives had fallen apart while living with alcoholics. They needed a self-help group to restore their own strength and hope. Families Anonymous was started for the same reasons by parents of chemically dependent adolescents. The two meetings have essentially the same format and philosophy. You will also find parents of adolescents at both meetings.

What happens at the meetings? When newcomers enter meeting rooms, people are quietly talking to each other. It is normal to feel scared and even ashamed because you are still uncomfortable and shy about things that are going on in your family. Someone may offer a hug. This may make you feel even more uncomfortable if you are not used to expressing feelings.

Parents will only hear first names at these meetings because everyone is anonymous. Also, the names of those struggling with drugs and alcohol are not even mentioned because they, too, are anonymous.

The meetings start with readings of basic principles, traditions, and inspirations common to the groups. Then there will be a speaker or a discussion topic. The newcomer will be able to identify with at least some of the stories told by others. There is no requirement to participate; you can just listen and remain silent. At the end of the meetings, group members usually form a circle and hold hands while saying a prayer.

Al-Anon and Families Anonymous are not religious fellowships, but they are spiritual. As stated in Al-Anon's *Information for the Newcomer*:

> *Members of any faith, or none at all, are welcome and we make it a point to avoid discussions of specific religious beliefs. The program is based on the spiritual idea that we can depend on a power greater than ourselves for help in solving our problems and achieving peace of mind. We are free to define that power in our own terms and in our own way.*[7]

Some parents find the association to a power greater than themselves so negative that they decide in advance not to attend these support meetings. A therapist explains this problem as well as what she offers as a solution:

> *Some parents react negatively to the suggestion that they must accept the concept of God in order to be part of Al-Anon or Families Anonymous or Nar-Anon. I know this is not true, but the words Higher Power can be confusing.*
>
> *I often wish that someone would write alternative language for people who believe in Eastern thought, or who are agnostics or atheists. I tell*

these parents that perhaps they could substitute a concept like the greater good, the human race, the good of mankind, a person they choose as a role model, their ideal self, or whatever. I don't want folks to turn off support because of difficulties with these two words. I often find myself needing to offer alternative options and have to respect clients' religious orientations.

There are no dues or fees to join Al-Anon, Nar-Anon, or Families Anonymous groups. There may be a basket passed around at the meetings, but this is only for voluntary contributions. This money is used by the group to pay rent for the meeting room and to buy the literature that is offered free to all who come to the meetings.

When some parents first are advised to seek out Al-Anon, Nar-Anon, or Families Anonymous, they think, "That's not for me!" Based on things they have heard from others or gleaned from the media, they might believe that such groups are based on, or modeled after, specific religious ideas that have caused them pain in the past. They might believe that they'll be forced or tricked into speaking about or confessing their own painful situation. They might believe that "Groups don't work," or "Talking doesn't work," or "Just listening can't help," or "Hearing other's problems is just depressing." With thoughts like these, they conclude that, "It might work for other people, but it won't work for me." They might believe that individual or group therapy with a professional has worked for them, and they don't want to try another kind of support group.

Parents may go to a single meeting and decide on the basis of something that happened there that they wouldn't go back. Perhaps the format of the meeting was confusing; perhaps there were only a few participants who didn't inspire confidence; perhaps it was held late in the evening and the drive was confusing; perhaps it didn't bring instant enlightenment. Or perhaps the expression of feelings by group members was too overwhelming. The mother of a teen addict who is now active in Families Anonymous describes her first experience at a Families Anonymous meeting and how the group helped her:

I had been going to therapy for several months when my son was using, but he refused to get an assessment. We didn't have leverage yet with court consequences to make him go, and without an assessment we couldn't send him to treatment. I was a wreck.

My therapist was helpful, but he was also encouraging me to go to Al-Anon or Families Anonymous. He said that he was helping me with some of my internal struggles over my son's situation, but I needed the support of other parents that could only be gotten at these meetings. He also told me that I would get ideas on what to do about my son, and I would get stronger in managing my life. I got so sick of him telling me this that I finally decided to go, just to get him off my back.

When I walked into my first meeting I felt shy and a little scared. People seemed so friendly and happy, and this isn't at all what I was feeling. When the meeting got going, I felt uncomfortable that so many people were open about their feelings, particularly their pain. Even with therapy for a few months, I had no feelings. I hardly knew what feelings were. I had forgotten how to talk like this in front of anyone, even my therapist. It seemed foreign to me. I was scared by it. It seemed that I would have to talk like this to fit in.

After the meeting was over, a woman came up to me and told me how Families Anonymous had helped her. She also said that I could come to as many meetings as I wanted without talking. She gave me a phone list and said I could call anyone I wanted because they wanted to support me. I felt no pressure to call or to come back.

The next week, I had more problems with my son, and I decided to call the woman who had approached me at the meeting. She gave me some ideas on what had worked for her in that situation, and she also supported me on an emotional level. It was wonderful.

I started going to that meeting regularly because I saw how it could help me. I am so glad that my therapist saw that I needed to see how other parents shared their feelings in order to get better myself. I also needed to hear other parents share their journeys and how they made progress. As time went on, members of the group were cheering me in my own progress, and that was really helpful to me.

My growth wasn't an overnight thing for me, however. It wasn't a quick fix from going to just a few Families Anonymous meetings. But I started to make progress, and I kept going. I felt so much happier. It was a process, and it is still going on.

The vast majority of people can get something very good out of Al-Anon, Families Anonymous, or Nar-Anon. Meetings are widely available in almost any location. They are free. They are anonymous. They help people.

Suspend your disbelief and go to several different meetings. Each meeting is structured a little bit differently (as well as being in different locations, at different times, with different participants). By shopping around for your "home" meeting, you can find the one that you get the most out of and that feels comfortable to you. Try to find meetings that have other parents in them, guaranteed at Families Anonymous, and often the case at Al-Anon and Nar-Anon. Attend a number of meetings of your chosen group, even if you don't feel comfortable and are not convinced the meetings will be helpful. If they are truly not for you, you can always discontinue them. The potential benefits, and the fact that they have helped so many, are worth giving them a fair chance.

Don't expect to feel clear-headed and "cured" after the first few meetings. It's taken a long time for you to feel this way; it will take time to heal. Do expect to feel better, over time, and to observe that others in the meeting will also be feeling better over time.

When you go to your first meeting, you will be told about a phone list of those who are volunteering to be called. Be sure to get this list before you leave and call people when you get home to help you with your many questions about what to do to help yourself and your adolescent.

Parents can find an Al-Anon, Nar-Anon, or Families Anonymous meeting in their communities by looking in the phone book for the contact number. If it is not listed, the Families Anonymous clearinghouse in Culver City, California, (800) 736-9805, will have information about meetings in the United States and Canada. More information is provided in Appendix A, *Resources*.

Additional action plans

In addition to going to support meetings, recommendations for parents include:

- Ask if there are student assistance professionals or prevention counselors at your teenager's school or if there is a counselor who focuses on substance abuse. Make an appointment to talk with this person about your concerns and ask how the school can help you. Jim Crowley's book, *Alliance for Change,* found in Appendix A, is an excellent overview of how schools and the courts can assist you in getting help for your teenager. Jim is president of Community Intervention, Inc., in Minneapolis, and they have a catalogue of other resources that many parents find helpful. They can be reached by calling (800) 328-0417.

- Parents who suspect their teenagers are abusing drugs or alcohol will need professional help to rule out drug/alcohol problems in a diagnostic interview and information-gathering process called an assessment. This process will be discussed in the next two chapters, but it will be important now to start asking around about where there are good assessment professionals. Ask people at your Al-Anon, Nar-Anon, or Families Anonymous meetings whom they have used.

- Start educating yourself further about alcoholism and drug dependency. Check Appendix A for recommendations. Three books helpful at this stage are Vernon Johnson's *Everything You Need to Know About Chemical Dependence* and *I'll Quit Tomorrow* and George McGovern's *Terry: My Daughter's Life-and-Death Struggle with Alcoholism.*

CHAPTER 2

Patterns of Development

There is an island of opportunity
in the middle of every difficulty.

—Anonymous

EVEN IF PARENTS UNDERSTAND the addiction process, they often have a difficult time when they try to figure out if their teenagers are harmfully involved with alcohol and drugs. This is because adolescent substance abusers often do whatever they can to conceal their use. Also, families can rationalize the usual signs and symptoms of problems with drugs and alcohol as being part of normal adolescence or some other problem or situation.

This chapter will examine what is normal in adolescent development, what can be considered problematic, observable behaviors that may indicate a problem with alcohol and drugs, how to sort out complications and confusing input, and what to do with information that is collected.

Myths of adolescence

In understanding tasks important for adolescents to master before moving into adulthood, certain myths can get in the way of reality about this age group.

Myth one: Adolescents are pathological

Many parents assume that strange or troublesome behaviors are to be expected in teenagers. This is a dangerous myth because it causes parents to assume that problematic behavior is normal. This can lead parents to shrug off problems in their early stages. Several parents explain their confusion:

> *My son was spaced out, wore army fatigues and earrings all over his body, and started hanging out with friends that looked just like him. I sort of thought he was just expressing his individuality in the strange way that*

teenagers do, so I didn't think much about it. I found out later that he was heavy into the drug culture, and what he was doing was part of that.

• • • • •

When we took our son for an assessment, the counselor said that he advertised himself as a drug user by the way he looked. We were shocked. We thought that all high school kids dressed this way. We had also gotten used to him disobeying rules and swearing all the time. We just accepted these behaviors as normal. We had decided that we were just too uptight as parents. That's what our son told us, and we believed him.

The great majority of teenagers are going to school every day, participating in school activities, and not harassing their parents with foul language. Also, they generally obey rules at home. They look more like the ads you see in the newspaper or in popular teen magazines. Parents can forget this. Of course, not all adolescents who dress in strange ways are drug users, and, conversely, kids who look like ordinary teens can also be drug/alcohol dependent. But the assumption that all adolescents look and act in ways that are pathological is problematic.

Myth two: Adolescents are homogeneous

Phrases that state "All adolescents do such-and-such" are problematic because they lead to overgeneralizing about the age group and overlooking problems. In fact, there is no more widely-varied group than this one. Any junior high school teacher can tell you that there can be a six-year span of biological development between an early-maturing girl and a late-maturing boy. To be told that a child is 13 says virtually nothing except for their age and probable grade placement.

Myth three: Adolescents are children

This is a dangerous myth because it overlooks the fact that adolescents are capable of reproduction, and they have strong romantic attachments. They are also capable of earning their own money, which can be used for drugs. In addition, they have greater freedom than they had in younger years, particularly if they can drive.

The myth that adolescents are children is particularly dangerous when it comes to sexual behavior as a result of drug use. Teenagers who drink or use drugs are much more likely than others to be sexually active. They can start sexual intercourse as early as middle school and with a greater likelihood of multiple partners.

Myth four: Adolescent growth is consistent

In fact, adolescent development can be quite inconsistent. Biological, sexual, emotional, and intellectual growth are not synchronized. Assuming otherwise can lead to false assumptions. As this mother explains, false assumptions can be dangerous:

> Our daughter was well developed and tall for her age at 14. We thought that her emotional maturity was at the same level. We weren't all that concerned when she started dating a 19-year-old. She said that the boys her age were too immature. We agreed with her.
>
> Unfortunately for her and for us, she was in way over her head. When she started doing things with this boy and his older friends, and got in trouble for underage drinking with him, we had to intervene. But she was really in love with him, so it was hard. It turned out that the guy was a drug dealer and he was using her. She was naive, and so were we. We thought that she was a lot more mature than she was because she looked so grown-up.

Myth five: Adolescence is transitional

Parents can overlook or minimize problematic behaviors by deciding to just wait out the years between 13 and 19. The father of a teen alcoholic describes this phenomenon:

> My son had friends I didn't approve of. He also had problems at school and with the police; I just sort of assumed that he would grow out of all this, and my wife agreed with me. After all, we sowed some wild oats when we were teenagers. We just needed to grin and bear it until he was 20.
>
> If it hadn't been for a suspension at school when our son was under the influence, we never would have taken him for an assessment. The principal told us that he needed it to re-enroll. We had made the mistake of not doing this earlier. He was assessed as a middle-stage addict. We wished that we had caught the problem sooner.

Normal adolescence

What is typical adolescent behavior? This is an important question for healthcare providers, teachers, school psychologists, and most certainly parents. It is also one of the major questions parents ask when they see their teenagers change. This father of a teen addict who was in treatment illustrates the confusion felt by many parents:

> Our daughter changed significantly over a short period of time. She was our oldest, and our first adolescent, so I thought that the changes must be due to hormones. It was hard to sort out how normal her rebellion was.

Adolescence refers to the psychological, social, and maturational process initiated by puberty. Puberty refers to a maturational, hormonal, and growth process that usually begins at age 12 or 13. What is normal in these processes?

When we are discussing what is normal, we first have to look at the problems with the word "normal" itself. Do we mean normal statistically? Culturally? In terms of how normal the person is as compared to a severe disorder such as schizophrenia? For purposes of this chapter, we will look at the perspective of normality as it relates to health. This perspective is elaborated upon in the scholarly and all-encompassing book by Irving Weiner, *Psychological Disturbance in Adolescence*:

> Health, in a positive sense, consists in the capacity of the organism to maintain a balance in which it may be reasonably free of undue pain, discomfort, disability, or limitation of action including social capacity.[1]

In using the phrase "reasonably free," this definition takes into account that some pain, some discomfort, some disability, and some limitation of action are part of the human condition. This definition looks at severity or matter of degree when assessing how normal certain conditions are, but, as this perspective suggests, it is not normal to be perfect.

The assessment of an adolescent for any problem is not easy. A school psychologist relates how an assessment is done:

> How much turmoil are these kids supposed to be in? This is an important question for me when a teacher or a parent refers a child for an assessment. What I have to look at are the normal developmental

tasks that an adolescent has to master to move into adulthood and if
something is getting in the way of these. In schools, we assess what is in
the way, and we draw up our Individualized Educational Plans to help a
kid move forward.

Developmental tasks

What is an adolescent supposed to accomplish before moving into adult-hood? Developmental psychologists and others whose research focuses on this area seem to agree that adolescents need to have significant changes in physical development, cognitive development, emotional development, social development, and in a sense of their own unique identity. These changes help them become adults.

Physical development

There are many physical changes taking place in youth between the ages of 13 and 19. Of most significance to overall development are changes in physical appearance and in the brain.

Body image is a very important issue for teens and a source of great anxiety. Girls are self-conscious about height, breast size, and weight. Much has been written about how they compare themselves to anorexic models and do whatever they can to look like these girls. Attaining the ideal weight might involve the discomfort of throwing up after every meal or not eating more than several crackers a day. Female peers can admire these behaviors, however, because they reflect control, self-discipline, and sacrifice. A teenage girl explains how she earned respect:

> *A lot of the girls at our school admired the fact that I spaced four*
> *crackers over the day in order to look the way I did. I had a tall glass of*
> *water for lunch and that was it. My friends would say things like, "Wow,*
> *how do you do that?" I knew they were jealous. It made me feel important.*

As pointed out in several articles in the *New York Times Sunday Magazine*, in a special issue called *The Troubled Life of Boys*, adolescent males are also struggling with attaining an ideal. In the article entitled "The Bully in the Mirror," Stephen Hall points out that teenage boys:

> *. . . tease each other, on a scale of casually nasty to obsessively cruel,*
> *about any perceived flaws, many of which involve some physical*

difference—size, shape, complexion, and coordination—and since adoles-
cent teasing begs for an audience, much of this physical ridicule occurs in
school.[2]

Hall describes the insecurity that results from this teasing and even raises the possibility that it is related to gun violence where teen males look for revenge, a way to get back at their tormentors. In her article "The Outsiders" in the same issue, Adrian Nicole Le Blanc describes behavior in a New Hampshire regional high school:

> *Bullying, here as elsewhere, is rampant. Even in a small town, sup-*
> *posedly safe environments like Peterborough, a 1994 study found, the*
> *vast majority of kids from middle school up are bullied by their peers. The*
> *shaming is sex-based, but the taunting is more intense for boys. . . .*[3]

Both of these articles note that the ideal physical body for adolescent males is that of the jocks. The outcasts do not generally talk about the teasing or their insecurities at home; to even admit their feelings would be an additional sign of weakness.[4]

While adolescents are preoccupied with their bodies and resolving their self-image issues, significant physical changes are also occurring in their brains and nervous systems. As discussed in the August 9, 1999 issue of *U.S. News and World Report* in an informative, reader-friendly article entitled "Inside the Teen Brain,"

> *Indeed, the brain inside a teenager's skull is in some ways closer to a*
> *child's brain than to an adult's. Still being forged are the connections*
> *between neurons that affect not only emotional skills but also physical*
> *and mental abilities.*[5]

Different regions of the teen brain are developing at uneven timetables and when puberty ends, the brain resembles that of an adult.

Cognitive development

The physical changes in the adolescent's brain include those that relate to cognitive development. Between the ages of 12 and 18, it is important for young people to develop an increased ability to think abstractly as opposed to only seeing the world in the concrete terms of a child. This cognitive development relates to the ability to generalize from experience, a helpful tool as you mature. Adults understand, for example, that if they drive a car off a cliff, they will crash and be killed. They also know from their experience, or that of others, that they have to avoid incarceration and how to support a family. Maturity means that you generally know how to live a responsible, productive life.

Social and emotional development

In terms of social and emotional development, the description of adolescents is as complex as the age group itself. A therapist with many years of experience with this age group describes their complexity:

> Adolescence can be described as the Age of Contradiction, the Age of Uncertainty, the Age of Measurement, the Age of Final Separation, the Age of Identity, the Age of Self-consciousness, the Age of Embarrassment, the Age of Competition, the Age of Dreaming, and the Age of Giving Up Dreams. All of this complexity is swirling around them as they develop.

In terms of emotional and social development, young people develop more of an inner sense of themselves—the task of individuation—as compared to others. They also develop a heightened sense of independence, an ability to function on their own. The latter is often referred to as mastering the tasks of autonomy and separation from their parents. It is also important that adolescents master the skill of developing healthy relationships, the ability to plan and implement productive use of their leisure time, and the ability to set, and achieve, realistic short-term and long-term goals.

Problems in social and emotional development often occur when teens have severe dependency needs, loose boundaries between their personalities and those of others and reality, or an inability to develop healthy relationships or appropriate intimacy. Professionals doing an assessment would also be concerned about profound sensitivity, mood swings that are debilitating, suspicious thinking beyond the norm for this age group, and a disturbance in self-image that is beyond the usual self-consciousness. As the normality of health definition offered in the beginning of the chapter implies, there would be concern if teens were less than "reasonably free of pain, discomfort, disability, or limitation of action including social capacity."[6] Severity of pain and other factors would limit their development.

Assessing social and emotional development is a challenge for any professional. A school psychologist who has been doing this for more than 25 years explains:

So much of our assessment is relative. We have to look carefully at behaviors and compare them to what is in the normal range. That isn't as easy as it may appear. Parents often think that we can make quick generalizations about their teenagers, but we can't.

John Glazer, MD, director of the Division of Child and Adolescent Psychiatry at the University of Rochester (NY) School of Medicine, states:

Adolescent assessment is especially complex because we try very hard to not see problems in isolation. For example, when we look at social and emotional development and try to assess psychiatric disorders, we also look at the possibility of substance abuse disorders. Research has shown that these problems often go hand in hand.

Substance abuse disorders and psychiatric disorders in adolescents are vastly unrecognized and only get worse if not treated. If parents are concerned about their kids, they need to get them to a team of professionals that includes an adolescent psychiatrist or psychologist. This is the first step for these teenagers to get the help they need in order to lead productive and meaningful lives.

More information about how to access professionals is in Chapter 3, *Assessment*, and in Appendix B, *Information and Help*.

Normal development and drug use

Parents can often feel that teenage drug/alcohol abuse is so common that it really isn't a problem. This is not true. If drugs are part of adolescents' lifestyle, there is a dangerous impact on their social, emotional, cognitive, and physical development. As a drug/alcohol assessment professional relates, drug/alcohol abuse is not normal and must not be minimized as a problem:

There is a problem with assuming that adolescent substance abuse is normal, and is something that every teen is doing. Making this assumption can cause two problems. The first of these is that parents can minimize substance abuse as a problem when they think that every teen does it. Although the great majority of teens do experiment with a drink or with pot, the great majority do not get hooked and have a lifestyle focused on using. Drug/alcohol abuse is not the expected teenage thing.

Secondly, by assuming that all kids get wasted and it's the normal teenage thing, parents can overlook the damage that is occurring to normal development when kids abuse drugs and alcohol.

Young people who start abusing chemicals at an early age, and then continue to use, lose a very important part of their lives. Substance abuse interferes with the maturation process. Another assessment professional comments on the unique challenge of assessment as it relates to development:

We have to look at developmental norms and if adolescents are moving along like they need to. When they are not, we look at how drugs might be the factor that is getting in the way. We then look at how drugs have served as a substitute for the healthier way that kids are supposed to grow. We ask ourselves how teens may be using drugs as a way to meet their developmental needs.

As discussed by internationally-known speaker on chemical dependence and intervention, Vernon Johnson, DD, in his book *Everything You Need to Know About Chemical Dependence*:

[Adolescents] use drugs to have fun, to feel better or stronger, to have more confidence on dates, and other internal reasons. Generally speaking, adults drink and use for more external reasons—the boss, the kids, the spouse, and the occasion. [For example,] many women blame a stressful life event such as death or divorce for their chemical abuse.[7]

It is important for parents to understand the internal reasons why drugs and alcohol are seductive in the adolescent culture. Teens who are abusing drugs and alcohol may be using them as a means to master the developmental challenges of the teen years in the following ways:

Using for a heightened sense of identity

Drugs and alcohol may make a person feel better about his or herself.

Drugs and alcohol may make a person feel important.

Drugs and alcohol may give a person a role.

Drugs and alcohol may be viewed as masculine or sexy or grown-up.

Using to improve relationships

Drugs and alcohol may function as status givers.

Drugs and alcohol may help a person gain acceptance.

Drugs and alcohol may facilitate transactions (making friends, giving courage, helping in seduction).

Using to increase autonomy

Drugs and alcohol may be used to symbolize rebellion.

Drugs and alcohol may be seen as "my decision."

Drugs and alcohol may be rites of passage.

Drugs and alcohol may be seen as forbidden fruits.

Using as part of leisure

Drugs and alcohol may be used as recreation.

Drugs and alcohol may prevent boredom.

Drugs and alcohol may be the focus of social events.

Using to avoid decisions

Drugs and alcohol may be used to alleviate anxiety about making decisions.

Drugs and alcohol may be used to postpone the challenges of adulthood.

This summary illustrates what parents are up against: drug and alcohol use is very seductive in the adolescent culture. Several things are important to remember, however. The first is that the majority of teens may experiment, but many do not abuse drugs and alcohol, and much less than a majority, about 10–15 percent of teenagers, are dependent on them. Unfortunately, the numbers of those abusing—and worse, those who are dependent—is in the millions. Also, even when teenagers are experimenting, they can be dangerous to themselves or others, particularly when they are driving a car or are experimenting with drugs like ecstasy or LSD that can scramble their brains in ways that can seriously affect their future.

It is important for parents not to minimize alcohol and drug use. An assessment professional explains how denial can happen:

I have heard so many parents regret that they just assumed that their kid was using to get friends or to fit in. They looked the other way, changed schools, or moved somewhere else. They thought their teenager would shape up.

Their kids may have started experimenting at parties like a lot of teenagers do, but then they got hooked. Now drugs and alcohol are at the center of their lives. The kids don't see this, however, and neither do their parents.

Another assessment professional relates how a parent learned the hard way:

I did an assessment in the hospital where a young man was covered with bandages because of a drunk driving accident. His parents were so mad at themselves. They had thought that their son just needed to find new friends and buckle down, be more responsible. They had lectured him about this, of course, and said that he would have certain consequences if he didn't improve his grades. But they said they should have taken him into an assessment to rule out drugs and alcohol as the cause of his problems. I always feel sad when I hear this. Their son could have killed himself, as well as other people.

Parents need to see how seriously they need to treat their teenager's drug and alcohol use. They tend to focus more on the symptoms and think of all kinds of excuses. It is important to rule out the bigger problem. They need to recognize that drug and alcohol abuse may be the answer.

Behaviors that result from possible drug abuse

Assessment professionals consider developmental norms when they conduct an assessment. They also look at certain observable behaviors that may indicate harmful drug or alcohol abuse. Knowing these in advance will help parents gather data for themselves so as to find the appropriate agency or professional for an assessment. Parents should also discuss these signs and symptoms with the person scheduling the assessment.

Just as there are warning signs for heart disease or diabetes, there are observable signs that teens are headed for danger with drugs and alcohol. One sign, by itself, may be meaningless, but several taken together are worth noticing and deserve a response.

Problems at school

Since school is required for teenagers, their behaviors in this environment give significant clues about possible drug or alcohol abuse. As stated by Jim

Crowley, president of Community Intervention in Minneapolis, in his book *Alliance for Change: A Plan for Community Action on Adolescent Drug Abuse*:

> Drug problems do affect schools directly. School staff members— from the administrators to the teachers to the nurses to the part-time office workers—are all on the front line; they see what is happening to students.
>
> School is also the place where a trained staff educates and nurtures young people and monitors their growth until age eighteen.[8]

Lower grades, lower achievement

Teenagers involved in drug and alcohol abuse or who are addicts/alcoholics will usually show changes in their grades and how they follow school rules. The mother of a recovering teen addict illustrates that these changes are relative, however, and must not be minimized if they are not dramatic:

> After we returned from a family ski trip, I got a phone call from my mother who wondered why her grandson was more withdrawn than usual. I told her that it was just adolescence. Or was it? On his last report card his grades had slipped. For the first time in ten years of school he had two Cs. Maybe he is worried about that, I thought.
>
> As I sat in my room thinking about his latest report card, I wondered again about the large number of absences in gym. "That was a mistake, Mom," he told me. "I switched sports and the old teacher kept marking me absent." I wanted to believe him. After all, he had always been trustworthy.
>
> The next grade report revealed two Ds and even more absences in gym. My husband and I then arranged a conference with the principal. She explained that our son was cutting gym right before lunch to have two free periods. Significantly, the two Ds were in subjects after those two periods when he was away from the school campus.
>
> When we finally had a drug and alcohol assessment, we learned that our son was getting high during those two periods. He didn't have the same level of concentration afterwards. That's why his grades changed.

Another mother of a teen addict talks about the progression of change:

> Our son had wonderful grades in elementary school and junior high, but when he got to high school they started to slip. We thought that he was having adolescent growing pains, and that we could just wait for things to get better. They didn't, and he ended up losing his whole junior year. We wished that we had paid attention before he failed everything. His decline coincided with his drug abuse. We found out about that later.

An English teacher reveals what often happens when teens are abusing drugs:

> We have a great school psychologist in our high school. She always wants to see how her referrals are doing in English. I can usually tell when a kid is abusing drugs by how they write papers. Their associations are pretty weak, and they argue with me about how things make sense when they really don't. All of a sudden they are these big defenders of creativity. Sometimes I even see pot leaves drawn in the margins of the stuff they turn in. It is pretty obvious what they are up to. They think they are being cool about it, though. They don't realize how much I know.

School attendance

Teens who are experiencing problems with drug and alcohol abuse will often have problems with school attendance. They often have unexplained absences during the day. In addition, many do not report to school at all, are excessively tardy, are suspended for rule violations, and are frequent visitors to the nurse, the gym teacher, or their counselor as an alternative to attending their classes. These types of behaviors can happen despite parents' best intentions. A mother of a teen addict explains how her actions did not guarantee positive behavior:

> I knew that my son didn't like school, but at least I could do my part and make sure that he got there. I dropped him off right at the door, and I even waited to see him walk in. What I found out later is that he would leave out another door and go to this empty house where he would get high with his friends.

The school psychologist who always checks with the English teacher reports on what she learns from others on the school staff:

> When I am gathering data in the junior or senior highs, I always check with the attendance officer. Then I visit the nurse to see her sign-in sheets and to see who shows up to hang out with the gym teachers.

If a school is lax about hall passes, certain kids just wander around. If you are high, or just under the influence, it is a lot easier to hide out wait-ing in a crowded nurse's office or wandering in the gyms, pretending some teacher has asked you to do something. The same goes for a counselor's office. Kids figure out how to wait, and even the counselor doesn't catch on. Some kids are just good con artists, especially when they are trying to protect their drug use.

Extracurricular activities

Teenagers who are abusing drugs can often start complaining at home that they no longer enjoy a hobby or a school activity. They may tell parents that they want to drop out. Sometimes they become ineligible from missing prac-tices or rehearsals. A recovering teen explains why he dropped out of an important activity:

When I was using, it was too much to have to get to practice in the summer before school started. I had been out partying the night before, and I wanted to sleep in. Also, I didn't hang out with my same jock friends anymore, and some of them even figured out that I was leading a double life. I didn't want to be around them. It was easier to just quit the team before I got asked to leave.

This is often very difficult for parents. They can go to great lengths to wake up their children and nag them to get to practice. Parents know that teens will have positive self-esteem if they can succeed in an activity. Unfortu-nately, if teens are abusing drugs and alcohol, that has become the center of their lives. They are hiding this from their parents, who are justifiably confused.

Disruptive behaviors

Teens who are abusing drugs and alcohol can become very disruptive at school. They can have defiance over rules, fight in the halls or outside, throw objects in class or in the lunchroom, engage in defiant littering, and get caught smoking cigarettes in the bathroom. Some students are involved in theft of school property or vandalism on school grounds. They may be brought to the attention of the principal because they are caught smoking marijuana on school property, dealing drugs on school property, or they arrive at school smelling of alcohol.

Parents are often involved in school conferences as a result of these disruptive behaviors. Some parents will be told that their adolescent needs to get an assessment to rule out drug and alcohol abuse in order to return to school following a suspension. The mother of an addict explains:

> Our son showed up at his first period class reeking of beer, and his teacher sent him to the principal. He had an elaborate story about how he happened to be drunk at 8:30 in the morning. It was such a ridiculous story that I don't even remember it now. What I do remember well, however, is that he was suspended. We were told that we could not bring him back until he had an assessment and followed through with the recommendations.
>
> I am so grateful that an assessment was required by his school. I was really in the dark about my son's using, but the assessment showed that he was an addict.

An assessment counselor explains that all parents are not as happy:

> Sometimes the only reason a teenager is brought for an assessment is because the school is requiring it. The parents are mad about this, and so is the kid.
>
> I take the parents aside and tell them that the school would not be doing this unless they had good reasons. I also tell them that they are lucky that the school wants to rule out drug and alcohol abuse. After all, it's life threatening. Their child could die.

Since the school day is a major part of adolescent life, it is an obvious source of data in terms of observable behaviors that may indicate problems with alcohol and drugs. Parents are encouraged to ask their children's counselor how their teenagers are doing in all aspects of their school life. Some schools even have tracking forms that they can circulate to all of the staff involved with a student in order to elicit comments about behavioral and academic strengths and weaknesses. Parents have a right to hear from schools about their adolescents.

Parents are also encouraged to ask schools to hold teens accountable. A principal describes how they can use parents:

> So many parents want their kids to be excused from the consequences of their actions. They don't see that their son or daughter is using them to

get out of something. Kids need to see that they receive consequences for breaking the rules.

Sometimes I have parents wanting to make sure that there will be consequences—and harsh ones at that. These are the enlightened parents. They know that [children need] to see that they made mistakes. This is how they learn.

Not all principals are so willing to help. As a mother relates, parents may need to exert extra pressure on their schools to hold their teenagers accountable for their behavior:

My daughter wasn't going to school, and I had suspicions she was using. But she wouldn't go to an assessment appointment either. She generally did what she wanted. Since the school didn't file truancy on her, she said that not going to school wasn't a problem.

I went to the superintendent to complain. I told him that if the school didn't follow up, kids think they don't have to come. I also told him that truancy may indicate drug abuse, and we need to acknowledge it in order for kids to have court leverage for assessments and treatment. He agreed with me and had a talk with the principal. Things changed. Now there are several kids in our high school that are in treatment getting help because the school filed truancy charges.

Changes with friends

Teens who are abusing alcohol or drugs will want to associate with others doing the same thing. Therefore, changes in friends can be an indication of problems.

Unfortunately, parents tend to confuse friends as the cause of their teenager's problems rather than a symptom of the real problem, drug or alcohol abuse. An assessment professional describes a common tragedy:

I have heard so many parents say that their teenagers would be okay if they didn't hang around certain friends or have peer pressure to use. What they don't realize is that their teenagers chose these friends, and they don't want to give them up either. The friends they associate with support their lifestyle.

The real tragedy is when parents send their kids to other schools, and their kids find new friends just like the old ones. Parents spend a lot of money on what they think will be geographic cures, and they don't work. Their kids are alcoholics or addicts. The money needs to be spent on treatment.

The mother of a teen addict who went to treatment explains what she wishes she had done:

We knew that our daughter was hanging out with kids who looked like bad news so we sent her away to boarding school. Thousands of dollars later she was kicked out for drug possession. We wished we had used the money to get an assessment to rule out drug and alcohol dependency. We finally did this, of course, but we could have done it a lot sooner.

It is important for parents to pay attention to whether their children have changed friends. Do the old friends come over like they used to? Do they call on the phone? Actually, phone calls can be a source of very helpful data. The mother of a teen addict describes what phone calls can really be about:

We started to get calls where we would hear a click as soon as we said hello. My daughter was a lot more interested in getting to the phone before we did, so she could answer first. We also had more calls after we went to bed.

One night my husband got up when he heard the phone ring. He heard my daughter talking low on the phone downstairs. When he walked into the living room, she put the phone down and started yelling about how we should respect her privacy.

What we found out later, of course, is that all the clicks were her drug-using friends. She would arrange drug deals on those late night calls.

Teens who are abusing drugs may not only change friends; they may also be more popular. Parents who bring their teens for assessments sometimes relate that their phones would always be ringing. They would be amazed at how suddenly their teenagers had so many new friends. This may be related to the fact that they are dealing drugs. It may also be that their teenagers are especially adept at finding places for drug- and alcohol-abusing friends to go to in order to get high without the watchful eyes of parents or the police. The phone calls are because a particular house has become a command post for illegal activity. The mother of a teen addict describes how their house was a command post:

*We found out in treatment that our son was the organizer of infor-
mation about whose parents were away and which houses were available
for kids to go to during the day to get high. Drug users would call our
house to get the latest place where they could break in and hang out.*

Problems at home

Teen drug and alcohol abusers try very hard to make sure they can continue
their lifestyle. Parents are often the last to know what these adolescents are
really doing. An assessment professional talks about her experience with
guilt-ridden parents:

*I see so many parents who struggle with guilt because they hadn't
known the truth about what their children were doing. I tell them what
good con artists these kids are, how devious, how manipulative they can
be, how much they coerce their brothers and sisters to lie for them. Actually, the more the parents are on to them, the more secretive they need to
be. Parents blame themselves more than they should.*

*But parents also need to be wary of what kids say. There are certain
behaviors to look for that might indicate problems. And parents need to be
just as clever as their children. What are they really doing? If parents
have suspicions of drug use, they need to go all out to get to the truth.*

Certain observable behaviors at home may indicate problems with drugs
and/or alcohol. These will be illustrated in the next four sections.

Physical changes

Teens who are abusing drugs or alcohol usually have physical changes, but
they will often try hard to minimize or cover them up. Over-the-counter eye
drops, for example, are used to cover up dilated pupils or red eyes from
using marijuana. These products may or may not work. Just having them
around, however, can be suspicious. Why are these teens suddenly paying so
much attention to good eye care?

Parents should watch for the smell of alcohol or marijuana in the house, on
clothing, or on their teenager's breath. They can also look for staggering or
stumbling, vomiting, slurred speech, and poor hygiene. A parent of a recovering teen addict describes the physical changes related to drug use:

Our son was usually so conscious of how he dressed, and he would shower every morning. When he started abusing drugs, he was really a slob. He didn't want us to comment on this either. He said we were too hung up about being clean. We found out later, of course, that this was part of his drug abuse.

Teens who are abusing drugs will sometimes have drug-related jewelry, hair clips, and tee shirts featuring drug-related bands or stars. They may also draw drug-related material on their clothing, books, desks, and their bodies. Many teen addicts, especially older ones, do not do this, however, so it is mentioned with caution. Parents should not rule out alcohol and drugs as a problem if they do not see these physical changes.

Mood changes

It is normal for adolescents to have mood changes, but these may also be indicators of drug and alcohol abuse. Several parents of substance abusers relate the impact of substances on their teen's moods:

Our son was much more volatile at home when he was under the influence of alcohol and drugs. One of his sisters would cry because she was so afraid of him. He was also much more aggressive with my husband.

· · · · ·

Our daughter was overly sweet and pleasant when she was drunk or stoned. This nice behavior kept me from seeing what was really going on.

Changes in the bedroom

You can tell a great deal about teens by looking in their bedrooms. Parents need to look for changes such as if their teens go from being neat to being a slob or even from being a slob to impressing everyone with how neat they are. A drug-free former teen addict explains:

A lot of my drug-using friends had parents going through their rooms because they were such slobs. I had drugs hidden in my stereo speakers, and I didn't want my parents to think that they had something to look for. I kept my room extra neat to keep them out.

Teens who are abusing drugs and alcohol will often spend more time in their rooms. The mother of a teen addict relates how changes and charm can go together:

> My son was very social with the rest of the family before he started abusing drugs, and then he would spend a lot of time in his room listening to music with the windows wide open because he said that he liked the fresh air, even when it was 30 or 35 degrees. We found out in treatment that he was smoking marijuana up there.
>
> Since we didn't really know about the sweet smell that marijuana had, we couldn't detect it, and the fresh air made our discovery even more difficult. He said that fresh air made him feel healthier. We believed him since he had also started to be a vegetarian and do other things like separate our trash. He said that he wanted to help protect the environment. We were proud of him because he seemed so sincere.
>
> When our son was in addiction treatment, he told us that those new behaviors were all part of a manipulation to cover up his drug use. Kids can be really charming when they are using drugs and trying to fool you. They want to protect their ability to get high. They admit to this in treatment. It really shows how strong addiction is. They throw away all their values in order to get high.

Teenage addicts will often abuse drugs in their bedrooms, and may offer these drugs to younger brothers and sisters while threatening them not to tell their parents. The mother of a teen addict relates how her younger son was drawn in:

> One of the most painful family groups we had in my 16-year-old son's treatment was when he confessed to encouraging our 10-year-old son to get high with him one afternoon. It was when I thought they were just playing Monopoly together in my older son's bedroom. His younger brother took some puffs of marijuana, but he was too scared to tell us because he knew that he had done something we would not approve of. Our older son apologized for this in a family group with tears streaming down his cheeks. He was so ashamed.

Parents need to be suspicious of what adolescents might be concealing in their rooms. An adult addict who has been free of drugs for years and is now a counselor in a teen residential treatment program, encourages parents to check their teenager's room when they are suspicious:

> When parents suspect that their teenagers might be using drugs, they need to do random room searches. I encourage parents to tell this to their kids, and that they lose their privacy once they are suspicious. I also encourage parents to tell their kids way in advance that if drugs are found, they will file charges on them and ask them to have an assessment. Parents need to tell their kids that under no circumstances are drugs allowed in the house. They need to do this to protect their kids, because they love them.

Missing items

Parents do not usually count their money or do an inventory of their medicine or liquor cabinets, but doing all of these could yield valuable data about possible teen substance abuse. Adolescents who are abusing alcohol or drugs will often steal money or jewelry from their parents. They will also drink alcohol from their family's liquor cabinets or refrigerators and steal prescription drugs. All of these behaviors are used to either feed their own abuse or to raise money to pay drug dealers. Three parents of teen addicts describe their experiences with missing items:

> Two years after our son went to treatment, he gave us an envelope with $200 in it. He had told us once that he had stolen money from us while he was using, but we never asked him about it. We never really noticed it missing, so we assumed it wasn't very much. We were amazed that it was $200.
>
> Of course, we were also amazed that just out of the blue he wanted to repay us. He said that he was taking responsibility for what he did, that was why. Giving the money back was part of his recovery. We were very proud of him. We hadn't raised him to be a thief. It was all part of his disease.

· · · · ·

> Our son used several thousand dollars worth of my wife's family jewelry to pay off his drug dealer. We realized this and filed on him. He was court-ordered for an assessment and treatment shortly after we filed.

· · · · ·

When we went to a counselor to help us with what to do about our daughter, she told us to start gathering data for an assessment. She also told us that if we noticed things that were wrong, it was important not to sweep them under the rug, but to recognize them for what they were.

We discovered that water had been added to alcohol in the liquor cabinet, and that money was missing. Our daughter was also coming in late from curfew and not obeying house rules. We called juvenile court and they told us how to swear out a warrant for her arrest as an unruly child. At the court hearing, we told the judge that we wanted to rule out drug or alcohol abuse. The judge required her to get an assessment.

Constant discipline problems

It is very difficult for parents to spend week after week giving consequences for violent or disruptive behaviors, broken curfews, messy rooms, or not following up on chores. However, once disciplinary problems have become so dominant that they are at the center of interactions, there is a possibility that drug or alcohol abuse or addiction is present.

Legal problems and legal consequences

Disruptive behaviors at school, in the community, or at home can, of course, result in legal problems. When these happen, they are additional observable behaviors that may indicate possible drug or alcohol abuse.

Legal problems can be especially difficult for parents. The father of a recovering addict explains what it was like to go to the police station:

One night I got a call from the police station because my daughter was caught entering an open window at a local university. She was drunk with some friends, and they were trying to bypass paying for a concert that was going on in the gym.

I'm a lawyer, so it was humiliating to have to go to the police station. Then I wondered if maybe the police were over-reacting. Don't all kids do something like this? When I walked into the station, I was confused and angry. My daughter was going to have a trespassing charge. She was sheepish when she saw me, but she was also very drunk. It was a very low moment for us.

As it turned out, however, the trespassing charge was really helpful to us. She had a legal consequence, and that helped all of us see that she had a problem with alcohol. She never would have broken in if she had been sober.

This father illustrates the importance of looking carefully at any law breaking or altercation with legal authorities as possible symptoms of drug abuse, addiction, or alcoholism.

In addition, it is important to note that this father did not try to have the trespassing charge revoked, and he saw how helpful the legal charge was to his daughter eventually getting help. More information about the important relationship between legal consequences and getting help is discussed in Chapter 3, *Assessment*.

High-functioning teens

Some parents can honestly say that their teenagers do not seem to have many of the problems we have listed, but, nevertheless, they suspect harmful drug or alcohol abuse. Two therapists relate their experiences:

In my therapy practice, I have known of kids who are athletes or performers in other school activities or creative kids who are risk-takers on several fronts, and their substance abuse goes undetected. They are actually abusing quite heavily, but their accomplishments are so amazing that the attention is more on those. Their peers report excessive consumption and blackouts, however, particularly on weekends. These are kids that have gotten in trouble with binge drinking, for example. One boy came close to losing his life from alcohol poisoning. These are also kids using party drugs like ecstasy, and their brains are in trouble.

· · · · ·

I have seen teens in my practice that are high-functioning in grades and school activities, and they are fairly compliant with home rules. They have gotten into scary situations on weekends with alcohol or drugs, however, and they pass out or are in accidents where everyone in the car was high or drunk. They get referred to me, and I sometimes find out they have serious substance abuse problems.

It is important for parents to rule out substance abuse problems if teens are high-functioning.

Dealing with conflicting input

Parents can be confused about what is going on with their adolescents. Many well-meaning people may provide them with possible explanations for problematic behaviors. Friends, neighbors, and therapists may say that teenagers are acting out to show their independence and that the teen's behaviors are a normal part of that process. Others may say that the teens are just trying to separate from their parents, and this is normal. Still others may say that all teenagers with psychiatric diagnoses like attention deficit disorder or depression exhibit the behaviors that parents are concerned about. These comments can so confuse parents that they become paralyzed. When this happens, parents stop asking for the help they need to rule out substance abuse that may exist simultaneously with other problems. The single mother of a teen addict describes how conflicting input hurt her:

> My son's grades had dropped, and he was no longer talking about wanting to go to the colleges that used to be so important to him. He had also dropped out of some activities at school that used to be a big part of his life. I had found some marijuana in the house, but he denied smoking it and said it was from his friends. A lot of my family said he was just experiencing growing pains and he wanted to be independent. I didn't want to over-react, so I decided to just wait it out.
>
> His behaviors got worse, and he ended up being suspended from school. The school principal said that he had to have a drug and alcohol assessment to rule out addiction as the cause of his behavioral problems. He went to the assessment, and we found out that he was addicted to marijuana and alcohol.
>
> I wish that I had called for an assessment appointment sooner. Just because you want to rule something out doesn't mean that you are over-reacting. But I was so confused, and so many people had different theories about how my son was normal.

Agencies and schools that focus on the possibility of drug abuse in students can often help parents move in a positive direction to get help for their drug-abusing teenagers. These outside agencies and schools do not always follow through in this way, however. Experts such as Vernon Johnson point out that, unlike adults, adolescents have many supporters—called enablers—who are willing to look the other way with denial, delusions, and rationalizations about the problematic behaviors that are often related to the drug-using lifestyle of teenagers. These enablers make it even harder for parents to sort out conflicting input and decide what to do next.

According to Johnson:

> The average chemically dependent adult might have as many as ten to twelve enablers—family, friends, in-laws, the family doctor, the boss, and maybe the court. In contrast, the average chemically dependent teenager might have 50 to 60 enablers—immediate family, grandparents, uncles, aunts, school personnel, church staff, law-enforcement officers, court personnel, medical staff, friends and parents of friends—all making it easier for the teenager to keep using.[9]

Even when parents are on the right track with understanding the signs and symptoms of drug abuse, enablers can sabotage effective intervention. The mother of a teen addict describes the difficult time she had with input from others:

> I wondered if drugs could be a problem for my son, but I didn't do anything about it except beat myself up about not being a good mother and, then, go to therapy to be a better one. I have since learned how typical this was and how self-defeating. It was my son that had the problem. He was the one who needed help.
>
> As time went on, my son's behaviors got worse. I started checking out what I could do to get help. I went to two different therapists and even got him to go to one of them. He refused to go back after two visits.
>
> He skipped school a lot, but I never got calls about his absences until he was flunking out and was being recommended for a special school for kids with behavior problems. I asked the police if he could be prosecuted for truancy and be compelled to attend, but they said that wasn't possible. My son loved that: he told me that the police only care if you murder someone. He thought he could get away with everything!
>
> When my son went to the special school, the problems with his behavior continued. I spoke to the principal on a number of occasions, saying I knew he had a drug problem. He said there was nothing I could do except toss him out on the street so that the justice system could get involved. He said it in such a way that a loving mother would never do such a thing.

I then told the company that he was working for that there was a drug problem. Actually, they had been suspecting drug abuse. But instead of requiring him to go treatment as a way to keep his job, they fired him.

My son's problems continued to get worse. I tried to take him to the doctor for drug testing, but, when we got there, he figured out what was going on and bolted out the door. The doctor said there was nothing I could do to get help.

When he turned 18, I kicked him out, changed the locks, and then, later, I moved. I hoped that the trauma would be enough to motivate him to go into treatment. Unfortunately, he moved in with another family that was focused on drinking and they just told me what a nice boy he was. Now he is living out of a van. He has no interest in getting help for himself.

This mother was never able to get help for her son, and he continues his destructive lifestyle. Her story illustrates the frustration felt by many parents who suspect drug and alcohol abuse, but are confronted with misinformation about what they can or cannot do. She also had many enablers who threw up their hands with an "Isn't it a shame" attitude described by Jim Crowley in *Alliance for Change.* According to Crowley:

Community members can react in much the same way as family members. They deny that young people are in trouble. They hide their own confusion, guilt, anger, and pain because they refuse to acknowledge the problem or because they believe that nothing can be done to improve the situation.[10]

In addition, what could have been helpful information to this mother about the court system was given with the implication that she would be an unfit, unloving mother if she "tossed" her son out on the streets. Insinuations like this undermine parental confidence and play on parental insecurities.

Another father, in another city, had a more positive outcome when a counselor and the court system responded:

I had so many people telling me that all the problems my daughter had were related to normal struggles that adolescent girls go through. I believed them for a while. They said that since I was a loving father, I just needed to forgive her and move on.

My daughter also said that she would never speak to me again if I contacted the courts. She said that there were horrible things that went on in the detention home, and she would kill herself if I sent her there. I didn't want to lose my relationship with her, so I caved in.

I started seeing a counselor who knew a lot about addiction, however. She told me that my daughter was just trying to pressure me to not hold her accountable for her behavior. If she ended up in the detention home, it was because of her illegal behaviors, not me. The counselor also told me the signs and symptoms of possible drug abuse. I felt much more confident of my perceptions, even when friends or family would say I was over-reacting.

She also told me how to use the court system to get help. She kept telling me that I was a loving parent because I was willing to make the difficult choices to help my child, even though she didn't want me to help her.

I phoned the police when my daughter ran away because I wanted them to pick her up. They said they were too busy with major criminals like murderers and rapists and that there was nothing they could do. I called my counselor, however, and she told me that I could swear out a warrant for my daughter's arrest on truancy, runaway, and unruly charges. I did that, and then the police went to get her. I even told them where she might be.

My counselor told me how the court system could work for me if I was persistent about it. I was, and my daughter was sent to a court-ordered assessment. She is now in court-ordered treatment. The treatment is a great opportunity for her to help herself.

This parent had a counselor who was able to point the way to the opportunities to bring about positive change.

Taking care of yourself

Parents who are gathering information about their children's behaviors need to surround themselves with as many parents as possible who do not minimize or rationalize what is going on. Such parents can be found at Families Anonymous, Al-Anon, or Nar-Anon. It is important to take advantage of the support that is out there.

CHAPTER 3

Assessment

Nothing in the world can take the place
of persistence.

—Calvin Coolidge

TEENS WHO ARE ABUSING alcohol or drugs will have problematic behaviors. On the other hand, these same behaviors may also be symptomatic of other conditions that need attention from outside professionals. When parents are suspicious of, or concerned about, their teenager's possible harmful involvement with alcohol or drugs, it is time to have an outside opinion about what is going on. A comprehensive, multi-factored assessment is necessary to rule out drug and alcohol, psychiatric, learning, and physical problems that may be impacting their teenager's lives. An assessment will also provide recommendations to parents for what will be needed to make positive changes for their adolescents.

This chapter will discuss how to access and select an assessment agency or professional to rule out drug and alcohol problems, how to arrange an assessment, how an assessment is done, what will be expected from parents, the range of what can be expected from teenagers, how a diagnosis is made, and what happens at an assessment summary conference. This chapter will also discuss what parents can do when their teenagers are not cooperative with the assessment process in order to maximize the chances that they will cooperate in the future.

Accessing and selecting professionals

Parents play a significant role in accessing help for their teenagers. A family therapist from Oregon who sees many troubled teens explains:

> *The role parents play when they are concerned enough to seek counseling for a teen is crucial. In our area, parents most typically start with family or individual counseling with someone who specializes in child and*

adolescent and family therapy. Alcohol and drug evaluation is not usually the primary focus. However, most therapists I know who see teens do ask routinely about substance abuse. In many cases, however, both teens and their parents underreport actual use. This may be because the teens want to hide what they are doing and, therefore, the parents are clueless.

I find myself asking a series of screening questions and asking parents for their ideas about what is influencing deterioration in behavior, mood, and change of friends, etc. Changes can also be occurring in terms of certain triggering events, so I ask about those, too.

I often remark that a certain profile of behavior sounds like the profile of someone who is abusing substances. I encourage parents to watch for signs of substance abuse, to do random room searches, to check their money and their medicine cabinets, and to do other things that will give more data. I also conduct random drug screens on their teenagers.

As a general therapist, I would see a huge difference in detecting substance abuse if parents would take a larger role in asking therapists to conduct a drug/alcohol abuse assessment or to recommend someone who can when their teenager is already seeing a counselor who may not be trained to do this. It would also make a big difference if parents would strongly suspect drug and alcohol abuse when teens start acting differently.

Drugs and alcohol are so easily available to teens these days. Because of this, parents should automatically be suspicious about the possibility of their kids' substance abuse. Such suspicion will result in a heightened awareness that may actually save their teenagers from harming themselves.

There are many qualified, credentialed assessment specialists who might be recommended to parents by enlightened health insurance providers, medical professionals, and mental health professionals. The best resource for selecting an assessment agency or professional will often be other parents in the same area who have taken their teenagers to an assessment. Parents like these are in support groups such as Families Anonymous and Al-Anon. The mother of a teen addict discusses the helpful advice she got from another parent:

My son had been very successful in school and in sports, with friends, everything, so when his attitude changed at home and his grades dropped, and he started missing curfew, I knew that something must be going on.

I had denial about drugs being the problem since I had not seen my son use, but I knew that family denial is a normal part of having an abuser in the home. I wanted to check out my observations with someone else.

I asked a friend whose son had had a drug problem. She was also attending Families Anonymous. She had told me how helpful it was to have other parents to consult with. She said that behavioral problems like my son had are related to drug use. I was doubtful that this might be the case, but my friend also recommended some places to call for an assessment. I told my insurance company that the problems might include drug abuse and they gave me a list including some of these places. I found someone working in one of them on a Sunday, and I was able to set up an emergency assessment for the next day.

I was really glad that I had thought to say to my insurance company that drug abuse might be a problem. The assessment agency looked at other possibilities as well, just like some other referrals would have done, but they were trained to do the additional evaluation of drug and alcohol use. We got our son to treatment for addiction right away.

What are the key elements in accessing help and selecting an assessment specialist? Consider the following:

- Be suspicious. Do not rule out drug and alcohol abuse as being the source of teen problems. Not seeing evidence of this means nothing. Teens abusing drugs and alcohol want to cover up their behaviors.

- Do not rely on asking teens if they are using. In fact, many professionals recommend that parents not even ask because this lets teens know that parents are suspicious. As a result, teens will hide their use and cover up problematic behaviors in more devious ways.

- Gather information. If possible, talk to other parents whose children have had the same problems. Parents will need to get referral ideas before selecting an agency or professional and talking to their HMO. If they do not have access to other parents or if they want additional information, the *National Directory of Drug Abuse and Alcohol Treatment and Prevention Programs* lists all assessment agencies, treatment programs, and state agencies that coordinate treatment and prevention programs. Call numbers relevant to you, explain your situation, ask how you can get help. If this catalogue is not in your library, call the Department of

Health and Human Services in Washington, DC, (800) 729-6686, to request a copy.

- Educate your health insurance provider. Tell them that you want to rule out drugs and alcohol in a comprehensive assessment. Ask if they cover the agencies and professionals in your area that you have researched. If not, ask how you can appeal in order to access these referrals.

- If your health insurance provider is not cooperating, find allies. Parents can complain to the human resources manager where they work, to their union, and even to their congressman. You will have more clout with your provider if you have allies.

What doesn't work

Parents have often learned the hard way that selecting an agency or professional to help them is not easy. As pointed out in a helpful resource for all medical decisions, *Working with Your Doctor*, by Nancy Keene, poor methods for choosing a doctor or another professional or assessment agency would include:[1]

- Picking someone out of the yellow pages. This is taking medical potluck. You could get an extremely well-qualified physician or professional or someone who lost privileges in a neighboring state for negligence and has recently relocated to your area.

- Calling the number seen on a television advertisement. These referral services are paid for by doctors or other professionals, hospitals, or agencies and are merely advertisements. In addition, most doctors or other professionals or agencies with good reputations fill their practices with referrals from patients or other physicians and do not need to advertise their services.

- Asking a local hospital for a recommendation. They will only refer you to physicians with admitting privileges at that institution or to other professionals who work there. The doctor or other professional may be excellent, or she may just be the newest person hired.

In addition, the best resource for selecting an alcohol/drug abuse assessment agency or professional may not be the parent's health insurance provider. These days, provider networks are often composed of only certain doctors with ties to only certain hospitals. This means that networks can function like doctors recommending others in their own practice. Health insurance providers may not have the assessment specialty parents are looking for, even though they tell you they do. Also, parents may not even have what are called substance-abuse benefits, an umbrella description for professionals who should know for sure how to provide assessments. The mother of an addict explains how she finally got help for her son:

> We live on a large ranch and have an HMO that covers many families like us in rural areas. We relied on their expertise when we thought our child was abusing drugs, but they sent us to a psychologist who was not trained to see the problem.
>
> Our son lied during therapy, and it wasn't until we found him in a coma in a pasture that we realized the extent of his use. We appealed the HMO's recommendation and eventually got to an agency out of the network that our insurance paid for. We hadn't even realized that our plan did not have substance-abuse benefits, but when we appealed, we got them. It took a lot of work on our part to get help, but we finally succeeded.

A father in a suburb near a large city has a similar story:

> Our son was having problems that we thought were connected to having moved so many times or the hormones natural to adolescents, so we decided that he needed counseling. We had first asked him if drugs were the problem, but he said no. Since we hadn't seen him use, we believed him.
>
> We called our HMO and told them what the problems were at home and with his grades. They gave us a list of mental health professionals and said they dealt with these problems. We had two therapists involved who believed my son when he lied and said we were the problem. Not once did these therapists examine his drug use or raise that possibility to us.
>
> It was a very difficult time for us because our son's behaviors were only getting worse. We had complained to our HMO when it seemed that our son was manipulating the therapists, so they sent us to a third person.
>
> Then our son was hospitalized when he was in a coma after a bad drug experience. We called his latest therapist, very upset. He said that he was glad that we knew about our son's using now because he had known for a while, and he was bound by confidentiality not to tell us. We were

furious. Our son could have died. None of the mental health therapists dealt with his drug use, which we found out later was extensive.

When we brought him home from the hospital, we told our HMO that we had confirmation that he was involved with drugs so we needed a new list of referrals. He finally got to an assessment agency.

We were just too trusting of professionals and of our son. We also did not realize that insurance providers are not diagnosticians. We had to rely on them for answers they were not capable of giving.

This father cautions parents to not rely on their children to be honest about whether or not they have a drug problem. Such honesty is rarely possible from those who are harmfully involved with drugs. In fact, it is normal for drug abusers or addicts to think that they are not having problems with using. Denial, delusion, and rationalization go hand in hand with drug abuse. Parents are in trouble when they believe adolescents who tell them they do not have problems despite behaviors that indicate otherwise.

In addition, getting teens to talk about their drug use can be a problem from the therapist or assessment professional's point of view. An adolescent therapist in private practice describes some complications with confidentiality:

Confidentiality is a difficult issue when we are trying to find out if teenagers are involved in substance abuse. Many teens are reluctant to discuss their problems openly, including substance use, when they believe that the therapist will tell their parents. This is a major dilemma for therapists, on many counts, when they hear that a teen is involved in careless, self-destructive behavior which therapists are not required to report under state law. These behaviors include sexual activity, drug and alcohol use, truancy, petty crimes, and intentions to run away.

Some of us make a point to discuss the limits of confidentiality in the initial session. We tell adolescents and parents that we are required to report child abuse and intention to harm self and others (suicide or homicide), but that there are many other behaviors that we are not required to report. I always ask the parents in front of the teen if they would expect me to report to them as the legal guardians of a minor any of the other non-reportable behaviors. In that way I get a clear contract established with both the teen and their parents. Parents often say they do not need to hear about drug use unless I think there's a problem.

I've handled situations where I do think there's a problem by telling the teen that I want to talk with their parent about my concern about how much trouble they're having and usually that includes a statement about my concern about drug use. I've had one parent back three times to appeal to her to look more closely and nothing happened.

In my area, at least, many family therapists are frustrated about parental reluctance to look earlier at the possible role drug use plays in their teen's manifestation of problems, or to heed warnings from therapists about drug use. Parents are much too trusting of their kids.

How can you tell when a drug abuser or addict is not telling the truth? An assessment professional with more than fifteen years of experience in the alcoholism/drug dependency field relates her experience with lying:

When parents ask me how they can tell if their teenager is lying or telling the truth about alcohol or drug use, I say that you can tell they are lying when their lips start moving. Parents question me on this, but I tell them that if teenagers are abusing or haven't been in recovery for long, they really have forgotten how to tell the truth. In fact, they don't even know the truth themselves. Their denial, delusion, and rationalization have been supporting their use, and they truly believe they do not have a problem.

Like health insurance providers, other medical specialists (such as pediatricians, internists, psychiatrists, or nurses) or mental health professionals (such as psychologists or social workers) may also be untrained in alcohol/drug abuse assessment. These are professionals who would be excellent to consult about many medical decisions, but medical schools and graduate schools do not always train their students to do alcohol/drug assessments.

Some graduates of these training programs may assume that if teenagers are abusing drugs, this is a symptom of other problems that need to be addressed first. These professionals tend to refer to individuals with a similar point of view unless they have had experience or training in alcohol/drug assessment, which is not as common as parents might assume. Counting on these individuals as experts in drug/alcohol problems is how teenagers do not receive help. As many parents relate from bad experiences, teenagers can die while lying to untrained therapists and getting away with it.

Arranging an assessment

When parents have selected an assessment agency or professional such as a psychologist or psychiatrist trained in addiction, they need to call for an appointment. Arrangements will be made for payment at this time. In Canada, the province funds all healthcare, including assessments, although there may be transfer payments between federal and provincial governments. One needs only to be a resident of the province to have free access, although some provinces may require a small co-pay. Some agencies/practitioners in Canada are private and will charge a fee. A Vancouver, British Columbia, youth counselor offers more details about accessing help in Canada:

> Some Canadian agencies that receive partial funding will charge on a sliding scale. Some extended health plans offered through employers will cover the cost of a counselor if the professional is a psychologist.

In the United States, parents will need to have knowledge of their insurance benefits, and what the co-pay or deductible is. Some assessment agencies and professionals will assist parents with this research. Some parents may also have concluded that their HMO will not cover the assessment. These parents need to inquire about the possibility of a sliding scale fee that will consider their income. Many private agencies offer a sliding scale thanks to community fundraising, United Way, or government funds that subsidize services. If teenagers are involved with the court system, they may be able to access court money to pay for the assessment.

The person answering the phone request for an assessment will ask parents for information about their adolescent's behavior problems. The more thorough parents can be, the better. Parents can refer to Chapter 2, *Patterns of Development*, and form a list of problematic behaviors to read over the phone. It will be especially helpful if parents have already gathered information about their teenagers from their school.

The assessment agency will usually request that parents bring their teenagers to the assessment appointment, but this is not always the case. They will also advise you on what to tell your adolescent. An assessment specialist offers some good advice for parents:

> I always advise parents to tell their teenagers that since there have been problems, they have made an appointment to get some help on what

to do to make things better. If it is necessary to talk about drug or alcohol abuse, it works best to say that it will be important to rule that out.

It would not be helpful to threaten or lecture your teenager with statements like, "I know that you have been lying to me, and someone smarter than you is going to come up with the truth!" That puts the kid on the defensive before they walk in my door. Also, that gives them time before the appointment to figure out ways to outsmart me. A power struggle gets set up, and a good assessment is almost impossible.

Dual-diagnosis issues

A comprehensive, thorough assessment by qualified individuals gathering data from many sources is necessary for an accurate diagnosis. As a family therapist who talks to many teens suspected of drug abuse notes, a comprehensive evaluation is needed to rule out a dual-diagnosis:

Parents should insist on a thorough psycho-social-biological evaluation, including a drug screen. Close attention needs to be paid to other comorbid conditions that are of equal concern to substance problems. It seems to me that depression, family discord, poor self-esteem, and social/peer problems so often accompany drug and alcohol abuse.

This therapist's advice reflects that of many working today in the addiction/alcoholism field. Dual-diagnosis is considered much more a possibility with today's youth than it was even several years ago because of the excellent research and reports on clinical experience that are highlighting the prevalence of co-existing or co-morbid conditions. A therapist shares her thoughts about the complexity of dual-diagnosis issues:

I'm not really sure myself sometimes which is the cart and which is the horse, but I do know that if drugs are a part of the teen's attempt to cope, that coping problem has to be addressed early on. In some cases, some teens are self-medicating with street drugs and alcohol against a mental health condition that has never been examined. I have seen some kids become well managed with medications when the possibility of a dual-diagnosis is part of an assessment. Sometimes, they have also become addicted to harmful drugs or alcohol while they self-medicate, however, so they need treatment for this in addition to their psychiatric medication. A comprehensive assessment will help to sort all this out.

Teenagers who do not cooperate

Unless substance-abusing teenagers have external pressure to cooperate with an assessment, they often won't—except if they plan on lying or if they are totally drug-free. Parents talking with an assessment agency on the phone may already know that their teens will not cooperate. Assessment agencies understand this. They will usually advise parents on actions they can take in order for an assessment to take place.

If teens, or adults, for that matter, are abusing drugs or alcohol, they have a denial, delusion, and rationalization pattern of defenses. They do not think they have problems with mood-altering chemicals or that they need to quit using. They do not want others to tell them to stop. They are not internally motivated to change their problematic behaviors by stopping their drug or alcohol use. Parents will usually have to apply external leverage through their own consequences or get the courts involved if teenagers will come to an assessment appointment. This is easier to do in the United States, however, since much of what is described in this chapter regarding the courts does not yet exist in Canada. A treatment specialist in Toronto comments on differences in Canada:

> Our legal system is quite different from that of the United States, so strategies such as parents charging youth with unruly or other charges don't apply, at least as of now as we begin 2000. Also, Toronto has the first Drug Treatment Court in Canada, but it is for adults, and there is no juvenile court like this.

Applying leverage with school and home consequences

Parents who wish to arrange an assessment will be fortunate if their teenagers have had negative consequences in school. Many schools require assessments to rule out drug problems if the student's misbehavior involved drugs. Some enlightened schools in both the United States and Canada will require an assessment or a visit to the school prevention or early intervention counselor even when they only suspect a drug-using lifestyle.

On the other hand, parents may need to ask for leverage from schools because it may not be offered. In fact, some schools may be resistant to this kind of cooperation because they are not sure if it is the school's role to help in this way. Schools may also be afraid that they will be held liable to pay for an assessment or treatment if they recommend it. They may not have funds for this, and parents need to make it clear that they are not requesting these funds. Doing so increases the chances that schools will then provide the needed leverage.

Leverage from home consequences could include loss of driving privileges if teens refuse to cooperate. In order to have driving privileges, they would need to cooperate with both getting an assessment and following through with whatever is recommended. This is a logical consequence if teens know that parents are worried about their drug or alcohol use, because they could kill themselves and others if they drive under the influence.

There may be other privileges that can be withheld to enlist cooperation. Many times, however, teens in trouble with drugs and alcohol will laugh off and disregard any of these efforts and refuse to cooperate. Court consequences may be the only thing that will work.

Applying leverage with court consequences

Substance-abusing teens who have the pressure from court consequences seem to generally have a higher rate of cooperation with an assessment. The mother of a now-recovering teen addict describes her frustrations and how court consequences helped her:

> I tried to get my daughter in the car three times to come to an assessment appointment. She wouldn't come, and I was furious. It wasn't until she missed her whole junior year, was dealing, and had possession charges from the court that she cooperated. I wish that we had had court consequences sooner.

The father of a teen addict relates to this anger and frustration and the importance of court consequences:

> We made our initial assessment appointment, but our son wouldn't get in the car. He said that this was ridiculous, and he would have nothing to do with it. We called the assessment agency. They said to come without him, and we did. They started us in a parent group to educate ourselves about addiction and how to hold our son accountable.
>
> We were getting stronger, and we knew that it was working when our son complained about the time we were spending by going to the group.

He complained that we were getting brainwashed. We were on to him, and he didn't like it. Then he ran away.

We were angry, but we weren't paralyzed by our anger like we had been in the past. As part of how much stronger we were, we called the police and they came over. We told the officer that we suspected drug use, and that there were probably drugs in the house. He brought in a book that he had in his car and showed us pictures of drugs and drug paraphernalia. We recognized some of the devices our son had in the house to assist him in his using and gave them to the officer.

Then the police officer asked us if we wanted to have a dog sniff out our son's room. We agreed to this. He found drugs, and we filed charges on our son for having drugs in our home.

Our son finally came home, and when he did he had a possession charge. The judge ordered him to treatment. It never would have happened if we didn't have court leverage. That policeman who searched his room saved his life. We were desperate to get help for our son.

Several other parents of addicts who went to treatment discuss the importance of paying attention to illegal behavior and making sure that this behavior has court consequences:

Our son climbed out of his window one night and did some vandalism in the yard while he was high with his friends. When he came in about five a.m., my husband was up, and he caught him. We saw the vandalism, and he admitted to it, so we took him to the police station to file unruly charges on him. He was violating our rules. We had learned in Families Anonymous how important it is to hold our children accountable for their behavior.

· · · · ·

We thought that our son had marijuana in the house, so when he left for school we called the police. The officers found it hidden in his stereo. When he came home, they also found some in his wallet. We decided to file possession charges and unruly charges. We had become educated about the importance of recognizing illegal behavior and not denying it. We are glad that we took action. The court required our son to go to treatment. He never would have gone without this. Court consequences saved his life. He is back in school and staying out of trouble. We are so grateful.

These stories illustrate that parents may have to play an active role in making sure that their children have legal consequences for their actions. Legal action may be necessary to protect children from hurting themselves or others. Legal consequences may be the only way that teenagers finally receive help for their drug or alcohol abuse or addiction.

The father of a teen crack/cocaine addict who is now in treatment talks about how the legal system helped his daughter:

> My daughter had legal charges for stealing checks from her mother and stealing her mother's car. We filed on her because we loved her, and we wanted her to get help.

> The charges were felonies, but they were related to using drugs. We have a special drug court in the Common Pleas division of our city court system, and it was through this court that she got an assessment. Then she was court-ordered to residential addiction treatment. She will have to serve jail time if she doesn't complete treatment.

> Before this, I looked the other way many times. She promised me that she would get better. She also threatened us if we talked about getting the courts involved. She said that she would get raped in the detention home, and it was a horrible place to be. We got scared. We know now that she was trying to intimidate us so we wouldn't follow through.

> We finally decided that she was a danger to herself on the streets, so being in jail couldn't be worse than killing herself with an overdose or in an accident when she was driving. We're glad we filed on her. The nice part was that she got help as a result.

The adolescent girl in this story, who is now in treatment, comments on how being involved with the courts helped her:

> I really want help for my addiction, but I am not strong. When the judge gave me a chance to get help, I was glad. I told my parents that I don't want to be like this. I don't like that I am on probation now, but it puts more pressure on me to stay in treatment and get help for myself. I need that. I wouldn't have gone to an assessment or to treatment on my own. I would have just continued the lying and manipulating to help me continue my drug-using lifestyle.

Court leverage can assist parents in saving their teenager's lives. It can be emotionally difficult for parents to file unruly charges on their teenagers for non-compliance to house rules and/or for not cooperating with the assessment or treatment process, but doing so is often the very thing that finally works. Several parents who attend Families Anonymous meetings for support explain how filing charges can help teenagers:

> *Kids don't want to go to the detention home, so when they have a choice of that or treatment, they often choose treatment.*

> *We can't beat our kids or chain them to keep them from destroying themselves, but we can call the police and file unruly charges. This is something that we can do.*

· · · · ·

> *What I have learned is that when I can detach myself, and not waste my energy on enabling, there are things that I can do to help my daughter and be responsible for my actions in the out-of-control situation. Filing charges was difficult for me emotionally. I felt that I had failed as a parent because I couldn't control my kid. But it is not that I failed; it is that my daughter's drug addiction was more powerful than I was. She needed that structure to rein herself in.*

An experienced counselor in an adolescent treatment program in Ohio relates how court consequences can be helpful:

> *Kids who have court consequences and a probation officer have a better chance at making an assessment appointment and then sticking it out in treatment. They have to think twice about acting impulsively and either not showing up or leaving.*

> *We wish that all parents had filed on their kids before bringing them in for help. They certainly had good reasons to. It is unusual for any kid in treatment not to have broken rules at home. They all should have unruly charges at least. And most of the parents could have filed theft and possession charges as well.*

> *The best way for parents to help their kids is to file on them. This gives the kids the structure to cooperate. So many kids bolt from assessments or treatment because they don't have to be accountable to the outside authority that the legal system represents.*

Because legal problems are so common with abuse and addiction, and because court consequences can be so helpful in providing the leverage for adolescents to get help, communities all over the United States and Canada are trying to respond. On both the adult and juvenile level, drug courts have been created in the United States to respond to individuals who are willing to admit to their felonies and desire help for the chemical abuse that led to the illegal behaviors. A similar option exists for adults in Toronto. Those who complete treatment, and submit to monitoring, can have their charges eliminated. A juvenile drug court assessment and treatment counselor in a large American city describes the intent of this special opportunity:

> *Teenagers certainly need to be held accountable for their misbehavior, but we do much better with preventing future legal problems if we also address their drug abuse. We hope to prevent the teens that come before the drug court from becoming violent criminals. We can require kids to get help, and this gives them incentive to follow through. They want to get the courts off their back.*

Many communities, like Cleveland, Ohio, and more than twenty of its surrounding suburbs, have also created voluntary courts separate from the drug courts to address petty juvenile crimes that seem insignificant in juvenile courts where judges hear about violent crimes and child abuse. These petty crimes include underage drinking, drug use, vandalism, shoplifting, truancy, curfew violations, or unruly child charges that have been filed by parents. The teens sit before volunteer judges who are lawyers called magistrates. These magistrates are from the teenagers' communities. Youth violators face such penalties as paying for damages they caused, cleaning up parks, painting fire hydrants, and doing other city projects. Some of the teenagers are sent for drug and alcohol assessments and treatment. Others are sent to anger management classes, school tutoring, and family counseling. If they comply with their sentences, their charges are erased.

In a recent study of 500 youth brought before this special court in Cuyahoga County (Greater Cleveland) over an 18-month period, only 12 percent have gotten in trouble again.[2] Juvenile court judges and others in the juvenile court system such as probation officers and referees "are reported as ecstatic."[3]

The local hearings were a solution reached in 1998 by Betty Willis Rubin, then the chief judge, after she learned that thousands of children accused of minor crimes never appeared before a judge. Detectives would investigate crimes, identify juvenile suspects and submit files for prosecution, all for naught. With no consequences, the youth had little reason to reform. The legal system was earning the reputation among teens as being a joke. Teens felt they could commit any crime short of murder and nothing would happen.

Drug abuse is significant among Cleveland teenagers and is yet another reason for court attention. Of twelve metropolitan areas nationwide where children are tested for drugs after arrest, Cleveland has the second highest rate, ahead of Los Angeles and Washington, DC. More than 62 percent of the children arrested in Cuyahoga County have evidence of drugs in their urine, according to the US Justice Department.[4]

Parents who have been helped by drug court involvement often feel that without this leverage, their children would not have received help. The grateful mother of an addict relates how drug court helped:

> My son was picked up for shoplifting, and he was also not going to school. He had problems before this, but he absolutely refused to go along with the requests my husband and I made to get him help.
>
> When a detective was assigned to his case, I asked if we could go through the drug court, which I had heard about from some parents at a Families Anonymous meeting. It worked out that we had a hearing where my son pleaded guilty to his charges, and then he got an assessment from a counselor who works for the courts. This is how he ended up in treatment. The drug court has a contract with certain agencies and they monitor how treatment is going. They also pay for it. It's a great use of our tax money.

Courts may also have a close relationship with schools, particularly if these schools have well-developed programs as alternatives to suspension. Jim Crowley, president of Community Intervention, points out:

> Parents should investigate if their school has an "Insight Program," an alternative to suspension program for kids caught using on school property or, in some communities, for kids caught using anywhere. These programs are an important community resource for parents, particularly when early intervention is concerned. Schools can work closely with the courts to help kids stay in school as well as to help them be accountable for their drug and alcohol using behaviors.

Parents need to investigate the options in their own communities to have court leverage. The amount of cooperation you can expect from law enforcement will vary according to what part of the country you are in. As this therapist from Oregon notes, however, there is still an advantage to using the courts, even if resources are limited:

> In Oregon, several years ago taxes were greatly reduced in a referendum, and this caused a huge decrease in the law enforcement services available for misbehaving teens. Parents can no longer expect police to follow up on a report that a teen has not come home or has run away. I hear stories from parents who come away discouraged when they call the police or the local detention facility asking for help.

> I do encourage parents to call the police about aggressive behavior, theft, and parties where underage kids are being served alcohol, or where illegal drug use is suspected, etc. I urge parents to file charges no matter what, and to let their kid know that they are calling the police. The very act of seeking the assistance of the police gets the message across that the parents intend to go outside the family and to facilitate serious consequences.

> Parents really balk at the idea of their kid getting charged. Part of this may be because Oregon teens over 15 are treated (i.e., punished) like adult offenders for many offenses that used to be handled in juvenile court (where there is a greater chance for rehabilitation). These teens can be placed in jails and prisons with adults. . .with some tragic results, I might add. Parents need to look at the situations in their own states and plan accordingly.

Different states have different legal consequences for drug and alcohol offenses, including rehabilitation. The Oregon therapist continues:

> In our state we do reasonable graduated punishment and rehab requirements for alcohol-related offenses. A minor in possession loses his license for a period of time, and has to participate in drug education classes. A first DUI leads to a mandatory 90-day loss of license and a mandatory drug and alcohol evaluation. Depending on that, the offender either does a diversion treatment (classes) or outpatient treatment, which allows the charges to be dropped in three years if there are no more offenses. Second and third offenses have more severe punishments and rehabilitation requirements.

Parents need to investigate the legal options in their own areas. If they do not exist, parents need to enlist other parents, judges, public officials, and community leaders and advocate for change. This is how parents can empower themselves and their communities. Judges such as Judith S. Kaye, Chief Judge of the state of New York, can become their allies. As Judge Kaye writes in the article "My Turn," in the October 1999 issue of *Newsweek*:

> Here in New York we now have fifteen drug courts that direct nonvi-olent defendants to strictly supervised drug treatment instead of prison, halting the door of drugs-crime-jail.

> We know that a defendant in court-ordered drug treatment is twice as likely to complete the program as someone who gets help on [his] own.[5]

The assessment process

Once adolescents finally arrive for an assessment, parents often have many questions about how the process works. An experienced assessment professional describes what happens:

> An assessment is like a fact-finding mission. I work with the parents and the teenager to get to the bottom of what is going on.

A second professional relates how information is gathered:

> I work to get as much information about as many life areas as I can. I need to see what is going on in school, at home, and what the adolescent has done with other agencies or professionals.

Parents need to be sure that assessment professionals are gathering data from a variety of sources, not just from themselves and their teenagers. A comprehensive assessment for adolescents will include an evaluation of their physical, social, intellectual, and emotional development, and how they are doing behaviorally in all aspects of their lives. This assessment is usually done in consultation with a team of professionals at an agency and in conjunction with information provided by outsiders. Parents make this gathering of information possible by signing releases of information so others can be contacted.

Assessment professionals will ask parents and teenagers to answer written and oral questions in order to obtain information about what has been going on. Parents are usually asked to describe how their teenagers have changed, and when these changes first became evident. Parents will also be asked about their knowledge of their teenager's drug or alcohol use and any consequences related to this use.

Assessment professionals will also want to know what it is like at home. The key here will be the teenager's problems with curfew, discipline, and rules.

A comprehensive assessment will also consider the teenager's mental health, and potential dual-diagnosis issues. Teenagers may have had a mental health diagnosis for years, and they may have been on medication. Assessment professionals will want to review past psychiatric and psychological evaluations and hospitalization records. They will want to know if the teenagers have been keeping scheduled appointments with their psychiatrists and if they have been taking their medication.

A team doing a comprehensive assessment will also want to rule out important psychiatric problems that might be causing behavioral concerns and/or complicating drug abuse or dependency. For example, if an adolescent has been hearing voices, when did this start? This is an LSD complication, but hallucinations also occur in certain mental health disorders. If he has threatened to harm someone, what is the nature of these threats and toward whom are they directed? There is a big difference in pathology if these threats are against individuals who have turned them in for using drugs or against random teenagers in their school. If he is paranoid, highly suspicious, when did this start? It is normal for drug abusers to be paranoid about being found out, but this is far different from a paranoid schizophrenic who thinks that men on television in a football huddle are talking about him.

Three general types of professionals who will be involved in an assessment are psychiatrists, psychologists, and counselors or social workers certified in chemical dependency. In good agencies, these professionals have a history of working together to provide the best comprehensive assessment possible for adolescents. Parents can expect that team members have discussed their teenagers and reviewed all the material that has been gathered in order to come up with an assessment. The assessment team will also tell parents to seek another opinion from another agency or professional if parents do not agree with the team's conclusions.

A parent's role

What is a parent's role in an assessment? As already mentioned, parents sign releases so that information can be gathered. Parents also play a major role in providing data, such as from the teenager's school, that will be used in making the assessment. Therefore, it is important for parents to be honest with whatever information is requested by assessment counselors. This is not as easy as it may seem. Two mothers explain how the assessment process can be uncomfortable for parents:

> When I brought my son in for an assessment, I was uncomfortable with the questions about the way I was living my life. I was divorced, and I had a boyfriend staying overnight a lot of the time. My son didn't like him, and I didn't really want to talk about that. I was worried that maybe this was the reason for my son's behaviors. My son talked about it with the counselor, so the truth eventually came out anyway. I felt embarrassed for not being forthcoming myself. Also, I had worried needlessly about the cause part. The counselor told me that a parent doesn't cause their child's addiction, no matter what they do, good or bad.

· · · · ·

> When we took our daughter for an assessment, the counselor wanted to know about our drinking. I was pretty uncomfortable about that, and so was my husband. He had started drinking too much over all these problems we were having, and I knew he wanted to cut down. But he didn't say anything about this, so neither did I. The counselor found out eventually since my daughter told her, but then we talked about how keeping secrets only teaches kids that it's okay for them to do the same thing.

A parent's feelings

Parents living with teenagers who are abusing drugs have painful feelings, which are discussed in depth in Chapter 5, *Working on Your Feelings*, and Chapter 6, *Harmful Consequences from Normal Feelings*. Common feelings during the assessment process are as follows.

Fear

Parents can experience fear during the assessment because they are part of an unfamiliar process with professionals they may not trust, who may not reflect their ethnic or racial neighborhood, and who may be located in an office or hospital that is unfamiliar and intimidating. In addition, parents may fear that they are going to be blamed for their teenager's problems. A therapist who works in an adolescent treatment program describes common fears:

When parents walk in, they usually feel that we are judging them for what has gone on with their child. It's as if they imagine a big F on their forehead, and that we are all looking at it.

No matter how much I think that I am reassuring them that they did not cause their children's addiction, it takes a while for them to really believe it, sometimes months.

They are embarrassed to talk about the fact that their children stole money or committed vandalism. I tell them that I know they didn't raise their children to lie, cheat, and steal. It's not like they looked at their babies in their cribs and looked forward to the day when these infants would steal from them. It's not like they wanted them to be addicts either. No, of course not. I get so frustrated at times with this big guilt trip laid on parents. If they had only been able to stop their kid, they would have. Outsiders don't realize how insensitive it is to blame parents. They do the best they can with what they know.

Vulnerability

The assessment process can cause parents to feel vulnerable. This is because questions will be asked about their own lifestyle and behavioral choices in addition to that of their adolescents. A father of a recovering teen addict illustrates this feeling of vulnerability:

When we brought our son for an assessment, I was not expecting that the counselor would ask so many questions about me. After all, I wasn't the problem. We were bringing him to get answers about what he was doing.

I learned later on that what the staff at the assessment agency wanted to understand is the effect of our son's behavior on the family. It was part of the diagnosis of his addiction to see what the family had gone through. They also wanted to know if there was a history of alcoholism and addiction so they could assess genetic predisposition or children of alcoholic issues. They wanted to get as complete a picture as possible in order to make the best recommendations to help us feel better. Our life had been very chaotic in the past year, and we needed recommendations to heal from that.

Guilt and shame

Parents often assume that they are being blamed when their teenagers have behavioral and/or drug and alcohol problems.

Parents often walk in the door of an assessment thinking that they have done something wrong. This is why their teenagers are out of control. Their shame and embarrassment comes from destructive assumptions in the larger society that if children of any age are not doing well, it must be the parents' fault. In-laws and other extended family members may also blame parents.

Parents who grew up in alcoholic homes are at high risk for blaming themselves for their teenager's use. This is because they grew up with an alcoholic parent who blamed others for use, and took on this blame. The mother of an addict relates how this impacted her when she took her son for his assessment:

> I felt really inadequate when I brought my son in. This was my only chance to be a mother, and I messed it up. Whenever questions were asked about what was going on at home, I assumed that the counselor was saying that I was the cause of his problems. I also felt inadequate about giving my perceptions about what was going on.

> When I started to get well myself, I realized that I read a lot into the questions that the assessment counselor asked. I had not really resolved a lot of issues from my childhood. I was still playing the old role that everything wrong was my fault. It was such a relief to let go of that.

Parents learn in treatment that they did not cause their teenager's addiction, but they do not understand this yet in the assessment phase. A parent who attended education groups once his adolescent began treatment speaks for many:

> When I first started treatment, I thought I would be the blame for my teenager's use. I learned that this is not true. He has a disease with a biological base to it, a compulsion to use drugs. I wish I had appreciated this sooner. I would have saved myself a lot of sleepless nights.

Surprise

Parents are often surprised and even shocked by information that comes out in an assessment. This father of an addict explains his surprise:

We were surprised at how far along our daughter was in her using, and it scared us. When she told us what she had done, we couldn't believe that she was still alive after all the things she had taken. We were so relieved that after three therapists who found nothing, we were finally getting the truth. We were so grateful that our daughter was actually sitting there and not in a grave somewhere.

These two parents of recovering addicts talk about their experience in the assessment process:

My husband asked me that night if I thought my son was lying [about his substance abuse]. We had not seen him use, and he had told us before his assessment that he didn't, so we thought that he was making all this up. Actually, we found out later that it had been even worse than what he told us that first time.

· · · · ·

When I heard my daughter's drug history in the assessment, I was floored. I knew she had been smoking pot, but I had no idea that she was using LSD, opium, and mushrooms. Actually, we found out later in treatment that it was even worse than that.

Anger

It is normal for parents to feel angry with their teenagers when the truth about their drug and alcohol abuse comes out. At the assessment stage, parents do not usually understand that they are dealing with a disease, and it is the disease that deserves the anger, not the addict. An experienced assessment counselor explains that anger is normal:

Parents are also angry at the hell that they have been put through because of the consequences from their children's destructive lifestyle. Good assessment counselors understand this anger and tell parents that it is justified.

Even greater, however, is the anger parents feel when their adolescents are not cooperating with the assessment. Parents speaking thus far had the advantage of their children being at least partially honest. This is not always how it happens. The mother of an addict shows how her son lied:

The first time my son had an assessment, he went because he wanted car privileges, but he lied about his behavior. I was too afraid of what he would do after we left the appointment to contradict him. The assessment agency was suspicious and put him on a no-use contract, but he started using that night and was hoping that he wouldn't get caught. When he went for drug tests, he taped a plastic bag of a friend's urine inside his pants. When he was told to go into the bathroom, he substituted that urine for his own. It worked twice, but the third time a staff member went into the bathroom with him and caught him. Then it all came out about what he was really doing. He had another assessment and entered treatment right away.

With what I know now, I wish I had brought a list to the first assessment with all his problems on it. I am a lot stronger now from going to Al-Anon, so he doesn't intimidate me anymore. He used my fear as a way to control me.

Parents are justified in their anger at their teenager's dishonesty and/or non-compliance during the assessment process. After all, parents are trying to get help for them, to prevent their death. The father of an addict describes the despair that is felt by many parents, as well as an unexpected outcome:

My daughter ranted and raved when we got in the car after our assessment. She blamed me that she was going to treatment and said she didn't love me anymore because I had betrayed her. She made no sense, but it hurt me anyway. I loved her, and I wanted her to get well. The way she was going, she was going to kill herself. The nice part is that she thanked me for putting her into treatment when she graduated.

Relief

Lastly, in addition to feeling vulnerable, blamed, surprised, and angry during the assessment process, parents generally feel relief. The last few months, and sometimes years, have been a nightmare filled with many painful feelings.

Making a phone call to set up an assessment appointment can require much courage and determination. Parents need to congratulate themselves when they take this important step. There is now an opportunity to end their personal nightmares, their personal roller coaster rides. Relief is on the way.

The assessment summary conference

Once the assessment team has completed a comprehensive, multi-factored assessment, parents will have a summary conference to discuss the evaluation. The team will have looked closely at diagnostic criteria for various mental and substance abuse disorders in order to make a determination of a diagnosis, or diagnoses, and also the range of alternatives for treatment.

Parents need to ask as many questions as they can during this summary conference to be sure they understand what is being said. They also need to be sure they understand the nature of abuse and addiction if their adolescents are assessed as alcoholics or addicts. This mother of an addict describes how not asking questions became a problem:

> *I was so intimidated by the assessment process that I didn't speak up and ask about addiction when I had my chance. For months into treatment, I blamed myself for my son's disease. If only I had been a better mother. I sat in guilt in every family group, waiting to be blamed. When I finally got the nerve to tell my son to just get it over with, he looked at me, really sad. He said that he told me in the assessment that it wasn't my fault. He had taken responsibility for his disease and his consequences like every recovering person does, but I didn't even hear him.*

Assessment recommendations

Recommendations for follow-up will be made as a natural consequence of whatever conclusions seem evident at the time of the assessment summary conference. These conclusions will be labeled diagnoses if professionals on the team, such as psychiatrists or others, are licensed to give diagnoses. The diagnostic criteria used in the United States, and by psychiatrists in Canada, will be those found in the *Diagnostic and Statistical Manual of Mental Disorders IV*, also known as the *DSM IV*, developed by the American Psychiatric Association. Teams of psychiatrists, other physicians, psychologists, social workers, nurses, occupational and rehabilitation therapists, counselors, and other health and mental health professionals revise these criteria frequently.

The medical term "diagnosis" is common in assessment or treatment in the United States because psychiatrists or other physicians have senior status on assessment or treatment teams in the traditional medical model. Other healthcare professionals such as psychologists or Licensed Independent Social Workers (LISW) or Licensed Professional Clinical Counselors (LPCC) are also licensed to give certain medical diagnoses.

Health insurance reimbursement in the United States usually depends on medical involvement. In Canada, where there in national health insurance and less dependence on the traditional medical model, there is not as much emphasis on the fact that a physician needs to be involved. Provincial reimbursement to agencies for assessments and follow-up services is not usually contingent upon a medical doctor being part of the team.

Complications with diagnostic conclusions

As much as it seems that an exact diagnosis or conclusion summary can be given as a result of all the work that professionals do in an assessment, this is not always how it happens. Addicts and alcoholics will often distort the truth about their use as part of their denial, delusion, and rationalization about their disease.

Assessment professionals work hard to get data about adolescents from outside sources. However, consequences may have been overlooked or minimized by parents and others due to enabling. Without observable consequences, a diagnosis is more difficult.

An adolescent addict in treatment after her second assessment relates what happened when she distorted the truth and her parents enabled:

> When I went to an assessment the first time because of some bad kid stuff at school, I thought I was just a recreational user. I knew I had made some mistakes with crack, but those days were over and there was no point in telling anyone about what had happened. I told myself that I was going to be able to drink since alcohol wasn't my drug of choice, and I didn't have consequences from alcohol.
>
> My parents didn't know about my crack use. Since there were problems in my family, they blamed my crack consequences on those. I told myself that I wasn't really lying about not having crack; I had decided I wasn't going back to it anyway.
>
> The people who did the assessment didn't get the truth, though, so I didn't get the help I needed from that first assessment. It wasn't until I went back to crack, left home, lived on the streets as a prostitute for a few years, and got busted that I finally got help. I wish I had been more open during that first assessment. I have a lot more to deal with now.

Another addict in treatment describes how he also left out details of his use. Fortunately, his mother had data that made all the difference in his getting help:

I came for an assessment because my mother caught me breaking promises about using fourteen times. As an example, I said I wouldn't use marijuana in the house, and she caught me.

When I had the assessment, however, I left out some of the painful stuff, the low stuff, because I wasn't planning on quitting and I was trying to make everyone think that my use wasn't really that bad. I left out that I would punch walls because I hated myself so much for the double life I was leading, the lies. I didn't want anyone to know that I would scrape my hand down the wall to make it bleed so I would feel the pain.

It has taken me a while to get honest with myself about the consequences of my using. This has been a major advantage to me of being in treatment. But I tried to manipulate everyone in that assessment. It would have worked if my mother hadn't had the list of those fourteen times I broke my promises.

Even though I was correctly assessed as an addict, the assessment would have been more complete if I had been more honest about my consequences. I would have been able to get the help I needed right from the beginning rather than waste all the time I did by manipulating the truth.

Another complication in the diagnosis of addiction is the nature of addiction for adolescents as compared to adults. Even if teenagers are dependent upon drugs or alcohol, this may not be evident at the time the diagnosis is given at an assessment, particularly the first time that an assessment is done.

Competent assessment professionals are cautious about giving a quick addiction diagnosis. It is not as easy as parents think to make this diagnosis. The diagnostic indicators of addiction in adults, for example, are not the same as with teenagers. An assessment professional explains some differences:

When I assess adults, I get concerned if they are drinking in the morning before going to work so they can steady their shakes. With teenagers, however, abusers will use before school as well as those who are dependent. There is a certain amount of status to use, and kids brag about it. Adults don't do this. Also, when adults hide their use from their spouse or other family members, there is more of an indication of a problem. When teenagers hide their behaviors from their parents, this is a pretty normal kind of thing that teenagers do about a variety of things in their lives.

Diagnosis options

The assessment team will try to conceptualize where an adolescent belongs on the continuum of use, abuse, and dependency. In the United States, more so than in Canada, the diagnosis is very important in accessing the appropriate level of care and the requisite reimbursement. Many health insurance plans, for example, do not cover residential treatment, so there may be more attention to the diagnosis because of the potential that it may not require a health insurance provider to pay and, therefore, to be involved. Some parents feel that health insurance companies look more for an excuse not to pay than to meet the needs of their teenagers and their stories have been given throughout these chapters. In Canada, since most facilities are publicly funded, one needs only to be a resident of the province to gain access.

In both the United States and Canada, there is an effort to match youth with the least intensive, least intrusive level of treatment intervention that will meet their needs. Assessment professionals will usually have one of three options to present to parents as a result of their comprehensive assessment. These options will respect the fact that more information about the adolescent may become known as time passes, and a different diagnosis may be made at a later time.

Not abusing or dependent

What this means is that the assessment team has been unable to find a match between the adolescent's behaviors and the *DSM IV* criteria or other standards that are used in making diagnoses.

Due to the life-threatening nature of addiction, assessment team professionals will have worked hard to verify this non-abuse/dependent conclusion through repeated calls to the adolescent's schools or other collateral sources to make sure that something hasn't been overlooked. Also, the team members will advise parents to get back to them later if there are legal problems, school problems, or behavioral problems at home or in the community that may be the additional behavioral data needed to point to abuse or dependency.

Recommendations at this level often include that since adolescents have had problems related to drug or alcohol use, they should not use these substances. They may be asked to sign a contract agreeing to this. In the Canadian Harm Reduction model, according to a Toronto treatment specialist, abstinence is at one end of the continuum, but it may not be required as often as it is in the United States. In both countries, adolescents at this level may also be recommended to individual counseling and/or family counseling to deal with issues that prompted the assessment. Schools in some communities may have High Risk groups for adolescents whose behavioral choices and life circumstances make them high risk for developing substance abuse problems. If parents find that their schools do not have these groups, they need to lobby for them. They are an invaluable resource to assist adolescents before things get worse.

Abusing

Sometimes adolescents are given an abuse diagnosis. They may also be dependent, but there is not enough data to justify this conclusion at the time of the assessment. The *DSM-IV* states that if someone is dependent, she has to have had repeated consequences for using for at least a year. Due to enabling, when these consequences are not applied, she may not be available as evidence in the assessment. An abuse diagnosis may also be given wrongly because adolescents have lied and conclusions from the test instruments or data from parents and others are not definitive enough to support a dependency diagnosis.

Recommendations at the abuse level will be similar to those given when it is only possible to make a non-abuse/dependency diagnosis. Parents will be advised to not enable while monitoring their teenager's behaviors closely. They will also be told to stay in touch with the assessment agency.

Another option at this level is to refer adolescents to harm reduction programs; these programs are more common in Canada than in the United States. A Canadian youth counselor in Vancouver describes how harm reduction programs work:

> *The belief of the harm reduction model is that substance use cannot be totally eliminated, but the harm related to substance use can be reduced. The goal of harm reduction programs is either the reduced use of substances or abstinence. Counselors help youth to identify and deal with harmful behaviors from using. Professional counselors provide factual information, resources, education, and practice in skills. They also help adolescents develop attitudes to eliminate harmful consequences of substance use.*

Similar programs exist in the United States and are usually called early intervention services or pretreatment. Professionals who work in a variety of settings, but who interface with youth, staff these programs. These could include programs in educational, health, mental health, child welfare, juvenile justice, or recreational settings. Assessment counselors may refer drug-abusing adolescents to these programs.

Dependent

When the diagnosis is dependent, some form of inpatient or outpatient treatment will be recommended. These options will be discussed in more depth in Chapter 4, *Treatment/Rehabilitation*.

Taking care of yourself

The *DSM IV*, listed in Appendix A, *Resources*, is available at libraries and bookstores, and the substance abuse section would be helpful reading during the assessment phase. Parents can be justifiably confused about the criteria used in an assessment. Additional assessment resources are also listed in Appendix A.

The best way for parents to support themselves during this assessment phase is to continue their education about addiction and to maintain their contacts at Families Anonymous or Al-Anon meetings. This support will be invaluable. As this father of two teen addicts explains, it is difficult to be in uncharted waters:

> *I don't know what I would have done if I didn't have my friends in Families Anonymous to bounce things off of and to get support. My wife and I were in uncharted waters about so many things. We were so glad to have the phone list of FA members. If one wasn't home, we called another. They helped us with so many questions.*

CHAPTER 4

Treatment/Rehabilitation

The winner is always part of the answer.
The loser is always part of the problem.

—Anonymous

WHEN ADOLESCENTS HAVE BEEN assessed as drug/alcohol dependent, assessment professionals will recommend some form of hospital, residential, or outpatient treatment, also called rehabilitation. This recommendation will be given as a way to help adolescents and their families address dependency upon mood-altering substances and the changes in lifestyle, attitudes, feelings, and behaviors that will be necessary to support the positive changes called recovery.

This chapter will discuss justifications for treatment, insurance and fee issues, and factors in selecting a treatment program, treatment options, the treatment process, and premature discharge.

The treatment process can be frustrating and challenging for parents because the denial, delusion, and rationalization that are part of drug/alcohol abuse and dependency continue to have significant impact. The winners are the adolescents and families who push through these difficult emotions and embrace change. Those adolescents and family members who do not will continue to have the same, or worse, problems than they had before the assessment process started.

Justifying treatment

When parents first receive recommendations for their adolescents to attend treatment programs, they often have mixed feelings. Several parents of addicts describe what they felt:

> *When we sat in the assessment counselor's office and got the recommendation for residential treatment, we felt that we had failed as par-*

ents. The only way our son was going to get well was to move out. We had a loving home and we were intelligent people. Why couldn't we just deal with this ourselves? We listened to the counselor, however, and learned what staff does and what treatment accomplishes. It was a lot more than we could do on our own.

· · · · ·

We had a difficult time putting our son in outpatient treatment because various extended family members told us that we were making too big a deal of his problems. They said that all he needed was a loving home. We wondered if we could just deal with this on our own. We weren't sure if we were doing the right thing when we brought him to treatment, but now we are so grateful that we did.

Both adolescents in these families went to treatment the first time it was recommended, but this isn't always how it happens. Two parents of addicts explain their regrets about not following through:

When I sat in the first assessment conference and heard about the need for residential treatment, I said to myself, no way. The agency had a treatment program on site, and I had seen the kids there. My son wasn't like them. He dressed better, and even though he had consequences from his use, they weren't that bad. I was sure that I could get information about the dangers of drugs from our family doctor and talk to him myself. And if he had to go to AA, I could just drive him and sit with him.

I turned down treatment that first time, but my son got worse, and we eventually came back for help. He had denial about the seriousness of his disease, but so did I. I was also taking responsibility for fixing him, which is impossible with an addict. I wish I had put him in treatment when it was first recommended because his problems were just more intense later.

· · · · ·

When we got out of the assessment conference, my daughter told us that she could quit on her own, and she would run away if we put her in the residential treatment program that was being recommended. She said she was sorry for stealing from us and running away and hitting her younger brother, but she would never do these things again.

We wanted to believe her, so we decided not to admit her. Within a week, she was right back to her old lifestyle, but we had lost our place on the list at the treatment program and couldn't get her in for several months. We know now that we were conned and intimidated by her, and we didn't understand the power of her disease. She sincerely wanted to change, but she didn't have a recovery lifestyle to substitute. She has learned that new lifestyle in treatment.

When parents struggle with justifying treatment, they often ask if it is necessary, if it is it cost-effective, and if it works.

Is treatment necessary?

Parents may have several reasons for asking this question. First of all, they may wonder if their children can just quit on their own. After all, it is obvious that drinking or using drugs isn't good for them.

Addicts and alcoholics who are not yet in recovery cannot think logically about their use and their consequences. They do not understand and accept their disease. As discussed in Chapter 1, *Use, Abuse, and Dependency*, they rationalize what they have been doing, often by blaming their parents for not giving them enough freedom. In addition to minimizing the problems they have had as a result of using mood-altering substances, they have no program of recovery to substitute for the attitudes and behaviors that accompanied their drug-using lifestyle.

Quitting like the parents did

Sometimes parents think that their children can quit on their own because this is how they turned themselves around. A father discusses this assumption and a common flaw in it:

I was pretty wild as a teenager, but when I got into my twenties and lost a few jobs and a girlfriend as a result of my use, I quit cold turkey. I knew that it was bad for me to party, so I just stopped.

When my wife and I brought our daughter to treatment, I didn't understand why she had to be there. She could just quit on her own like I did. What I realized, however, is that I quit later, and it is a lot different when you are a teenager. Also, I may have been an abuser, not an addict.

I realized how powerful her disease was, and that she had a lot of denial about her consequences. That isn't the way it was with me when I quit.

Other roads to recovery

Lastly, parents may wonder if the comprehensive type of treatment or rehabilitation that is most commonly recommended for adolescents is necessary. This treatment usually involves a team of counselors, social workers, psychologists, art therapists, recreational therapists, psychiatrists, and, in residential programs, teachers. Their teenagers will have individual therapy, group therapy, art therapy, be required to attend Alcoholics Anonymous (AA) and/or Narcotics Anonymous (NA) meetings, and the whole family will have family counseling. Isn't there an easier road to recovery?

Other roads to recovery do exist. Adults who have chosen them will argue about their success, even though the research on this conclusion is limited. These alternatives are discussed in books like *The Recovery Book,* by Mooney, Eisenberg, and Eisenberg, listed in Appendix A, *Resources.* The authors discuss such alternatives as acupuncture, hypnosis, aversion therapy with drugs and/or electric shock, and cognitive skills development therapy.[1] They also discuss Rational Recovery (RR) and Secular Organizations for Sobriety (SOS), both of which reject what they call the spiritual approach to AA.[2]

These approaches are generally not recommended for adolescents who are assessed as dependent on drugs and alcohol, a later stage than abuse. They depend upon a certain level of motivation that adolescents do not have. More importantly, however, they do not address the complexity of the adolescent and the loss of normal development that has occurred as a result of their alcohol/drug dependency. This complexity is addressed in the more traditional treatment that is commonly recommended for the adolescent age group.

Is treatment cost-effective?

Parents asking this question want to know the cost factors if they go ahead with treatment. They first need to consider the costs if they do not.

Costs without treatment

At the most, costs without treatment include the possibility that adolescents might die of overdose or in driving accidents that also kill others. At the least, there are the psychological, physical, social, emotional, and intellectual costs to adolescent development when it is halted due to drug/alcohol abuse and dependency. There can be unwanted pregnancies, AIDS, or venereal diseases that add complications for the future. There may also be financial costs. The mother of an addict who eventually brought her son for treatment comments on money misspent:

> The assessment counselor at our first assessment recommended treatment, but I didn't want to spend the money because I thought that boarding school would work just as well. We spent money on that, but he was kicked out for using drugs. Then he hit a tree in our car when he was drunk, and we had a repair bill. Our insurance company raised the premium on our car. He was involved in some vandalism a few months later, and we had a lawyer. He also stole some of my jewelry to pay off some drug debts.

> We spent a lot more money keeping him out of treatment than we would have if he had gone. We had no idea these things could happen. We would have saved money if we had gone ahead with treatment when it was first recommended. My son had promised us that he would improve his behaviors on his own, however, and we had believed him. Now we understand how powerful his disease was, and how he needed treatment to help him.

Paying for treatment

The costs of not following through with treatment need to be considered when addressing how the treatment fees will be paid. In Canada, fees are provided through the national health plan, although some provinces require a relatively small co-pay. In the United States, many health insurance plans, including Medicaid, provide funds for some form of treatment, outpatient being the most common.

When parents do not have existing, or adequate, insurance funds, it is important to ask employers or employee unions to lobby for these funds and to seek other allies. It may also be possible to have court funds pay for treatment. The treatment agency itself may have a sliding scale based on family income as a result of United Way or community fundraising. See Chapter 3, *Assessment*, for related material on how to procure funding.

Parents need to be prepared for the fact that once their children enter treatment, it is not a short-term process and the expenses will add up. Many adolescent programs require that teens and their families be involved in one-to-two years of continual care from residential to structured outpatient to maintenance in weekly aftercare. Teens with this long-term involvement are more likely to maintain abstinence and non-using behaviors than those who have a less intense regimen.

Treatment versus passage of time

Treatment is lengthy on even the adult level, according to Marc A. Schuckit, MD, in the informative book *Drug and Alcohol Abuse: A Clinical Guide to Diagnosis and Treatment* (which is listed in Appendix A). In discussing whether or not the rehabilitation efforts are likely to yield better results than the passage of time alone, and thereby justify their cost, he writes:

> *A definitive trial of treatment versus no treatment is difficult to carry out because of the problem involved in insuring that men and women in the no-treatment group do not enter care anywhere else during the study period and because of obvious ethical considerations.*[3]

He goes on to quote studies showing healthcare costs accrued by individuals with substance-related disorders before treatment as compared to after treatment:

> *One such study carried out in the 1990s with over 4,000 individuals demonstrated that post-treatment healthcare costs were 24 percent lower than comparable costs for untreated individuals.*[4]

Similar studies are done on the adolescent level with the cost of adolescent treatment compared to other costs, such as those to the justice system when juveniles with substance abuse disorders do not receive treatment. On both the adolescent and adult level, these cost comparisons have led to an increase in drug courts and other measures to encourage treatment. Untreated substance abusers repeat their appearances in the justice system and drain the national and state budgets with funds needed for incarceration.

Outcome statistics

Parents considering cost benefits of treatment need to ask treatment programs for outcome statistics. The quality programs will have these in their files to justify their funding from donors, private foundations, and the government, and as part of what is required for their ongoing accreditation. These statistics will indicate how adolescents who have completed the programs do in comparison with those who dropped out. They will illustrate the continued costs parents will have if their teenagers are not successful in treatment or if they never attend at all. They will also help parents see if treatment programs help adolescents overcome their denial about their drug/alcohol abuse.

> Our son was in a lot of denial about his use when we entered treatment, but I also did not understand the power of this denial and how it complicates the treatment process. I was expecting a fix, a cure, within about three weeks. We are still in treatment a year later.

> Now I understand the disease, but I certainly didn't at the beginning. I was glad that I asked about program graduates. Knowing that kids succeeded gave me hope.

In better programs, outcome statistics will measure quality of life issues such as adolescents remaining in school after treatment, being free of the legal system, and continued sobriety. When these are favorable, parents can have increased confidence in the treatment program.

Does treatment work?

Answering this question is relative to the assumptions behind what is expected in terms of outcomes. Information about cost benefits illustrates that treatment works as compared to the costs if it is not tried.

Treatment benefits for adolescents

Adolescent treatment programs should be able to provide parents with outcome studies on such things as their clients' involvement in the justice system, attendance at school, and behaviors at home. These outcome statistics will help parents see how the programs impact teens attending them. Programs will also have abstinence rates, but these alone are not reliable because it is through behaviors that teens indicate whether or not they are leading a drug-free lifestyle. Also, drug tests can be unreliable because of the devious ways addicts can guarantee positive results; parents would not have absolute knowledge of the reliability of the treatment program's drug tests.

Many recovering alcoholics, addicts, and treatment professionals will say that treatment always works, because even if the addict or alcoholic doesn't get well at that particular time, they are nonetheless changed. An addict describes how treatment helped him even though he relapsed:

> I ran away from treatment the first time and was on the road for about a year. I had learned that I had problems related to my drinking, and even though I tried to bury these by using, it wasn't the same as before treatment. In a way, treatment ruined my drinking. I am glad I finally realized it and came back to get help.

Treatment benefits for families

Family members also change as the result of treatment programs if they make a decision to take advantage of the education and therapy groups that are offered. Four parents of teens who were either kicked out of treatment for violating major rules or who ran away relate how treatment made them stronger:

> I am much stronger in parenting skills than when we started treatment. Even though my son ran away, I know what to do. I am also a better parent to my other children.

· · · · ·

> In knowing more about this disease, I know that it is not my fault. Treatment also taught me how to reach out for help and not feel ashamed. Even if my daughter doesn't get well, I have learned how to ask for, and receive, help from others.

· · · · ·

> I have gained the ability to remove myself from the roller coaster of my son's use. With the reinforcement I will receive as I work my own family program of recovery, I will find the strength to carry on no matter what my son does.

· · · · ·

> In family treatment, I learned how I have been a codependent and an enabler and that I can no longer fix my child. I have become aware of how he has manipulated me in the past, and I have learned ways to avoid having this happen in the future.

These comments illustrate that parents receive benefits from treatment no matter what happens to their adolescent addicts and alcoholics. Siblings and grandparents also benefit from family treatment as they work on understanding addiction and the feelings they have about it.

Factors in selecting a treatment program

Selecting a treatment program can be overwhelming, as one mother describes her confusion:

> When my husband and I sat in the assessment conference, the counselor recommended several options for treatment. We were confused about what it meant for our son to be an addict, and we had never heard of these programs. We never thought that our son would have to go to these kinds of places, because we had a good home. We didn't even know what kinds of questions to ask to select the best treatment option.

Gathering preliminary information

After assessment agencies recommend specific treatment programs for adolescents, parents need to call them for fee and insurance information, a description of their services, information about their waiting list, and a summary of their outcome statistics. In addition, parents need to check out the reputation of those programs with other parents at Families Anonymous, Nar-Anon, or Al-Anon meetings. They can also ask their pediatricians and staff in the Employee Assistance Personnel (EAP) programs at work if they have heard about the reputation of these treatment programs.

Accreditation issues

Parents can also ask each program if they are certified in their state or province and, in the United States, with the Joint Commission on the Accreditation of Healthcare Organizations (JCAHO). The latter is the most highly respected healthcare accreditation organization in the United States and has strict guidelines for high-quality healthcare, including substance abuse treatment. Treatment programs are visited at least every three years for a three-day survey of these guidelines in order to maintain accreditation. They are also required to correct deficiencies immediately. Parents can ask treatment programs what their JCAHO scores were in the last survey, if they had deficiencies, what they were, and what they have done about them.

Common elements in quality treatment

Parents can feel relieved when recommended treatment programs have state certification and are in good standing with JCAHO. Most of the better programs are. In addition, insurance funding usually falls to these programs because they deliver what health systems or health service providers are looking for in quality treatment.

Elements in quality treatment include that adolescents be treated with respect for their disease—not as bad or crazy and in need of punishment. Also, treatment plan reviews are required, staff treating clients have professional addiction and/or mental health certifications, confidentiality is respected, a professional tone prevails, and competent pediatricians and psychiatrists treat both medical and psychiatric issues. Parent education is required as well as family therapy. Safety and medication issues are addressed for adolescents with conditions such as epilepsy and for those who are struggling with mental health disorders.

The leadership in state-certified and JCAHO-approved programs comes from qualified, credentialed specialists, and staff-to-client ratios that are more than adequate. In these programs, the schedules for clients are balanced with multiple treatment modalities designed for the clients' benefit and not the convenience of staff, and there are expectations for adolescents' behaviors which are enforced. In addition, JCAHO requires recreational therapy, school in residential programs, healthy meals and snacks, and a safe, clean, handicapped-accessible site where treatment is given and Twelve Step (AA or NA) meetings are a part of treatment.

JCAHO programs are required to respect, and program for, all sexual orientations, ethnic and religious backgrounds, races, and socioeconomic levels. These are intangibles, however, and parents need to study the atmosphere in treatment programs to assess whether or not the intent to respect all clients and be inclusive is actually practiced.

When state-certified and/or JCAHO programs are not available in a particular area, all of these are factors to look for in treatment programs.

Since adolescent drug and alcohol dependency treatment costs time and money for adolescents and their families, it is important to look at treatment programs critically before making a final choice of where you will place yourselves and your teenagers. The quality treatment programs have nothing to hide; they will welcome your questions.

Treatment options

Assessment agencies will recommend residential or outpatient treatment for adolescents. The more restrictive or less restrictive options are considered according to certain criteria such as whether or not adolescents are of danger to themselves or others. Clinical care placement criteria have been developed by adolescent clinical service providers and the health service providers and governmental agencies that fund treatment.

Clinical care criteria

Clinical care criteria standards for placement may differ slightly across the United States and Canada, but they generally follow certain criteria that are evaluated by treatment teams before and during inpatient or outpatient care. Following this treatment team evaluation, decisions are made for initial placement in a particular level of care, for continued stay in that level, and for discharge.

Health insurance providers and governmental funding agencies will hold treatment programs accountable to a close evaluation of these dimensions. They will talk with treatment staff about them and ask treatment staff to use them to justify one form of treatment over another.

Clinical care criteria used by managed care for placement of adolescents with substance abuse disorders in Cuyahoga County (Cleveland), Ohio, are an example of the type of criteria that are used for adolescent placement across the United States and Canada.[5] The managed care criteria in Cuyahoga County have been adapted by adolescent service providers in that area, a partnership system that is also used in many places across the United States between private and public heath providers. Questions for each criterion are examples of those asked during clinical care placement evaluations:

- **Acute intoxication or withdrawal potential.** Are adolescents at high risk of continuing to use drugs and alcohol despite the need for withdrawal?

- **Physical health conditions and complications.** Are physical health conditions sufficiently stable to permit participation in outpatient treatment, or do the risks of drug use or pre-existing conditions such as pregnancy or diabetes place adolescents in imminent danger of serious damage to physical health?

- **Emotional/behavioral conditions and complications.** Are adolescents having thoughts of killing themselves or others, or is there a recent (within the last 30 days) history of uncontrolled aggressive behavior that endangers self or others? Is the risk of endangering self or others manageable in an outpatient setting, or are behaviors sufficiently chronic and/or disruptive so as to require 24-hour professional intervention and separation from the current environment?

- **Treatment acceptance/resistance.** Is there an agreement to cooperate and attend all scheduled activities by adolescents and their parents, or is there total refusal by an adolescent to participate in treatment despite other forms of leverage (such as court involvement), motivation, or support? Is there non-acceptance or resistance to the severity of the problem despite serious adverse consequences/effects on health, family, work, or social life?

- **Abstinence potential.** Are adolescents able to maintain abstinence with outpatient treatment, or do they require a more intense level of therapeutic intervention?

- **Recovery environment.** Is removal from a volatile and/or non-supportive living environment necessary to allow stabilization and recovery skill development? Are parents or caregivers able to provide consistency of participation necessary to support outpatient care?

- **Family/caregiver functioning.** Do family/caregivers exhibit the generally consistent ability to define and maintain the appropriate rules and expectations in the home? Is family/caregiver use of mood-altering chemicals problematic? Are they willing or unwilling to assess their chemical use and follow through with recommendations including treatment?

Treatment program staff evaluates these criteria carefully when they are making decisions about inpatient or outpatient care for adolescents. A treatment program counselor describes the evaluation process:

> *The longest staff meetings in our treatment program are those when we are evaluating the appropriate level of care for a client. We first do*

*this after an assessment is done. We ask questions based on the place-
ment criteria and decide the most appropriate level of care. We continue
this process frequently as we observe how our adolescents and their families are doing in treatment. We want to be sure that we are meeting the
adolescents' needs in the best way possible by matching them to the most
appropriate level of care.*

Parents and the criteria

These categories and questions will be swirling around parents while they
are in treatment. Knowing them helps parents to appreciate, for example,
that the recovery environment in their home and their caregiver functioning
are evaluated for continued stay or discharge from a treatment program. Parent education and family therapy are required for parents to help develop
the skills to follow through. How parents participate in their own treatment
will be important. The father of an addict explains how important participation can be:

> *When we brought our son to treatment, I knew he needed help, but I
> was surprised that family treatment also included a focus on me. Our
> son's counselor told me that the insurance company was questioning con-
> tinued stay because I wasn't attending parent education groups, and I
> missed some family treatment groups as well. I didn't know that my par-
> ticipation was that important.*

The criteria also illustrate that treatment teams and health insurance providers are looking at a variety of dimensions with adolescent alcoholics and
addicts to justify continued stay or discharge from a particular inpatient or
outpatient level of care. Treatment team meetings are going on 24 hours a
day. This can be very significant for parents, as one mother relates:

> *I was so grateful to my son's treatment program for all the work they
> put into helping us. My son was a handful, but so were his parents! We
> had a lot of questions about what was going on, and we never imagined
> all the work that went on behind the scenes. My son's counselor told me
> about all the treatment planning meetings, and our health insurance rep-
> resentative told us how impressed she was with the depth in the reports
> that were written about our son's progress.*

Disagreements about placement

Due to monetary constraints in the current healthcare market, adolescents are usually recommended to outpatient care when they first enter the treatment continuum. Parents are often told that their children need to fail at this level in order to qualify for the more intense residential care or hospitalization.

Parents may not agree with their insurance provider, drug court, or other government agencies about the level of care these organizations are willing to fund. Parents may need to appeal these decisions. This can be a frustrating process, and it is helpful to have allies. Several parents who were successful in arranging the coverage they wanted relate how they got allies:

> *Our son had psychiatric issues in addition to his chemical dependency, and he was carving up his arm to let it bleed. Our health insurance provider said he was appropriate for outpatient care. My husband and I were incredulous. I complained to the manager of health insurance benefits where I work. He was able to get the company to change its mind to allow residential treatment.*

• • • • •

> *Our health insurance provider only offered two weeks of outpatient treatment for our son, so I appealed. I raised a stink about it and said they really didn't understand addiction. I also complained at work and the office manager lobbied for me. We eventually got more treatment, but the staff at the agency had to give reports every few days to justify continued stay.*

An appeal process also exists with state, court, or provincial funding. Parents may not be as successful in these appeals as they had hoped.

Many parents in the United States have complained to their senators or congressmen about their struggles with health insurance providers. Those who are new to these frustrations are encouraged to join these public complaints. This could result in legislation for change.

Regardless of the level of care, there are common elements to quality treatment that are discussed earlier in the chapter. There are also certain commonalities to the treatment process that parents go through for themselves.

The treatment process for parents

For parents, the treatment process can be overwhelming and frustrating. There is a slow pace to change, adolescents continue with the same behaviors they had at home, and parents have to listen to these problems in phone calls from staff or in family groups. Addiction to mood-altering chemicals remains strong, and adolescents continue to have denial.

Starting treatment

When parents first start treatment with their adolescents, they can feel relieved, grateful, and confident at the same time that they feel resentful. Parents of addicts relate common stories of what happens when treatment begins:

> I was really glad that my son was getting help, but I really resented him for everything he had done, all the hell we had gone through. Then I was told that I had to attend a parent education group for six weeks on Saturday mornings, and I was furious. That was my one day to sleep in. I wasn't the one that needed help. I wished that the staff would just take my son, and I could pick him up in six months. I needed a long vacation from him. That's how I would get well, not in a parent group.

> • • • • •

> I knew my son needed help, and I was really upset at the beginning that all we could get was outpatient treatment. I knew he needed more. I suspected he was using, but the treatment team could never catch him. It was a very difficult time for us. Then he fell apart enough that residential treatment was justified.

> • • • • •

> When we first entered treatment, I continued to get criticism in my family that if I hadn't treated my son the ways I did, he wouldn't need to be in treatment. They also said that if I kept this up, he was going to leave my home when he is 18. They were sure that he didn't have a drug problem because he had told them so.

> I ended up not speaking to the family members who said this stuff, even though that was painful. My husband and I just needed to circle the

wagons. We needed to keep the focus on following through with what my son needed.

Time showed that we were right because my son relapsed. He did have a drug problem. My family was conned by him. Maybe they will realize this some day.

• • • • •

When I first walked into family group with four other families and our son was sitting there with a counselor, I felt nervous and uncomfortable. No way was I going to say anything. Then I watched my son sitting there. It's like he was saying that we were all full of it, he didn't need this, and get off my back. I felt frustrated, like we were talking to a wall. I thought for sure that this was going to be a big waste of time.

• • • • •

Our first Sunday visit in residential was horrible. Our son was self-righteous and blaming and really abusive of us. We had been attending parent education, however, and we weren't willing to take this anymore like we used to. The staff person on duty told us we should tell him that if the behaviors continued, we would leave. They did continue, and we left. We felt so empowered. Those small steps of being different from the past were very significant to us.

By the next week, our son figured out that if he was going to have visitors, he had to act in a better way. These were some of the lessons he was learning; his behaviors had consequences.

• • • • •

Our daughter said nothing in our early family groups, and she would just sit there with a smirk on her face. It was infuriating. And then we would drive home and be met at the door by my mother who was babysitting our other child. She would be all happy and say, "Well, how did it go?" She couldn't understand at all because she had a family like the Waltons. Somehow that made it even worse. We were really lonely.

• • • • •

The beginning of treatment was really hard. Our daughter was an outpatient, but we were having so much difficulty with her that we decided to let her live nearby with her grandparents. They were enabling *her, and she was manipulating them to think that we were the ones with the problem. It didn't matter to us because we were getting some relief.*

Then our counselor told us that as long as we continued this arrangement, we were saying that we had no power with our daughter, she was stronger than we were. She was also using alcohol where she was and not getting consequences. I didn't know what to do. I didn't want my daughter home.

My husband and I talked about it, however, and we decided to tell her that she could no longer stay with her grandparents. She had to come home and live within our rules. We were scared about what would happen.

As soon as we told her, the power shifted. She was no longer in control. She even had the nerve to complain that we only gave her two days to make the switch before we picked her up. This was ridiculous because it had only taken her a few hours to run away from us in the past.

When she complained, I realized that even though I thought I was in control by not having her around, I really wasn't. The jig was up, though, and she knew it. This was when we first started getting well as parents. We were learning how to take our power back in our Saturday parent education group. It was working.

Parents making changes

As adolescents are struggling in accepting that they need to be in treatment, parents often get excited about the changes they can make in themselves. These changes are difficult at first, however. Four parents describe what they worked on and what happened:

At the beginning, I could hardly talk in our parent education group or in family group without crying. I was so overwhelmed by my feelings. What really helped in parent education was to get rid of some of the baggage from my childhood. I really worked hard on that.

Our parent group counselor kept saying that the past is the past, and we can't let it paralyze us in the present. I started to learn that I was doing the right things. All the belittling stuff about me that I heard in my childhood wasn't true now. As soon as I started to feel more confident about that, things started to change for me. There was so much other stuff that had been getting in the way from my past, and it was such a relief to get rid of it. I was so proud of myself for my changes.

· · · · ·

At the beginning, I was just going through the motions. Then I heard someone talk who came to our parent education group. He told us how he started treatment with his son that same way. I started to understand that I needed to work more on myself, just like our speaker did.

What I learned most is that I thought I could control more than I could. I was tearing myself up inside to make my son change, and he was acting the exact opposite of everything that I was telling him to do.

I had a problem with my anger, and I learned how I played a part in setting up the power struggles with my son. I would have had a heart attack or an ulcer if I had continued with what I was doing. My son would have really finished me off. I have worked on not having road rage in my house. I came to see how out of control that was, and that it didn't work anyway. Also, it was a form of enabling because it took the attention off my son and put it on me.

· · · · ·

When we first started treatment, I was really upset when I heard that I needed to work on myself. No one seemed to appreciate that I had worked so hard to help my son. I was so glad to get him out of the house and into residential treatment. All I needed was a time away from him. Otherwise I was fine.

I just sat in my stuff in my first parent education group. I resented that the counselor was so happy. She said that things could change for us like they had for her. Yeah, right! She didn't really understand my situation and me, and I would never learn anything from her.

At the second parent group, she read this book to us about a runaway bunny and how the mother was always there to catch him. At first it was cute, but as she read on, I just started to cry. I really let myself go. I sobbed. Someone had to leave the room and find more tissue because we ran out. This is the way it was for me. I had tried so many times to help my son, and he had done the opposite of what I had told him.

I started to get well that day. I realized how much I couldn't control my son by rescuing him, and how I was enabling. The parent group counselor knew a lot more about me than I thought she did. I thanked her when the six weeks of group were over, but I told her that I didn't want to hear any more bunny stories!

· · · · ·

It really helped me when I started to learn in parent education about the signs and symptoms of the disease and how they applied to my son. We were real confused at the beginning about what was normal teenager stuff, and he had been enabled because of this. He was used to getting his way. He didn't think that he had to have consequences for his behavior.

When we started to learn and get better, it was exciting. We felt proud of ourselves. Our son couldn't manipulate us. It was almost funny to see him pull some of our extended family members in so they could enable him. He was desperate to stay in his old behaviors. They would use the same excuses for him that we did. Then they saw how he was using them. They were learning, just like we were.

What is really good now is that we are all on the same page and our son doesn't have enablers to turn to like he did in the past. This means that he gets better because he has to be honest and take responsibility for his choices. He can't get away with things like he used to.

Painful phone calls and family groups

Adolescents struggle with old behaviors in treatment until they learn to substitute new ones. The using lifestyle involved lying, manipulation, aggressiveness, abusiveness, and a disregard for the feelings and property of others. Also, if adolescents still want to use, they may relapse while they are in treatment. It is painful for parents to receive phone calls about their children's misbehaviors or to be reminded of them in family groups. Parents who have been in treatment describe common experiences as teenage substance abusers struggle:

When we got phone calls from staff about things that our daughter had done that were negative, it was really difficult for me.

After the first two days in treatment, for example, we found out that she had opened the door of a car in a park where the treatment group had gone on an outing. She helped herself to a pack of cigarettes, and the staff caught her. They decided to file an entering charge on her to hold her accountable for her choices.

When I got the call from her counselor, I felt helpless, hopeless, and worthless. All the encouragement we were giving her wasn't making her change her behaviors.

I was scared by the fact that even though she was in treatment, she was continuing to do the same things she would do at home. On the other hand, I was relieved that now the treatment program had to figure out how to handle her. I was ready to learn some new ways. What we had been doing wasn't working.

· · · · ·

The most frustrating times in treatment were to find out in our outpatient family group that our son had relapsed again. I kind of knew it because he started being mean to his little brother, or he was getting caught in lies like he used to, but it was hard to listen to the word relapse and to listen to yet another contract that he would be on to turn himself around. This whole process was just going on so long. I wanted it to be over.

· · · · ·

When we came into residential, our son kept the same using behaviors he had before. We were so frustrated by the time and money we were putting into all of this and he wasn't getting it. We would be in family group and he would look at us with these endearing eyes. We knew he wasn't paying attention to the counselor. It was as if she was saying blah, blah, blah, for all he cared. I had an impulse to smack him.

You just don't know what to do anymore. We thought seriously about pulling him out because of the time and money we were spending, but then he started to turn around.

I think that what I have learned most is how strong an addict's denial is. Knowing about the disease has really helped me hang in there to keep him in treatment.

· · · · ·

When our son relapsed and went from outpatient to residential treatment, I had a really hard time in family group. I wanted to have hope for

him and to encourage him, but the words wouldn't come. I felt there was
no hope. It was a lonely time for me. I got a lot of comfort from staff
reminding me about the power of the disease.

· · · · ·

Family groups were hard. We were really down about the slowness of
our son's growth and almost pulled him out of residential treatment. But
then the reality hit. What would we do if he weren't there? At least there
was some structure, something we could hold on to. And then our son did
start to improve. Now he has made enough progress to move to outpatient.

We are glad that we didn't drop out. We also know that if he totally
fails, he will have to leave and that will be his consequence, not ours.
Then we will use the court system and maybe that will help him want to
have a better life.

Premature discharge from treatment

Some parents have to deal with their adolescent's premature discharge, however. This is because adolescents can be kicked out of treatment for not making progress despite repeated attempts by staff to help them. They can also be discharged prematurely if they have violated one of the major group rules. These rules exist to keep the treatment site drug-free and to maintain a safe and secure atmosphere that is conducive to treatment.

When adolescents first enter most quality treatment programs, they learn that the use of mood-altering chemicals on site is not allowed, physical violence and threats are not allowed, and sexual stimulation and intercourse are not allowed. Treatment programs that enforce these rules find they are making headway in showing addicts and alcoholics in their care that they cannot violate the rights of others. They are responsible for their choices.

Parents can feel frustrated, angry, and confused when their children are discharged prematurely due to lack of progress or because they break major rules. After all, these are the very behaviors their children came to be treated for. Shouldn't they be allowed to stay? Is treatment only for healthy kids?

On the other hand, when parents begin to understand the importance of not enabling, they can accept the discharge. A parent relates how she changed and how this helped when her daughter was discharged prematurely:

When I got the call that my daughter was being discharged for fighting, I was depressed and frustrated. I knew that the treatment program had worked hard to help her with her anger, and I was upset that she hadn't learned what to do. I knew she was in denial about her problems, and her coming home was going to make it even harder for me.

She cried on the way home and said that she knew she had been wrong. I was glad that she had been held accountable for what she did. Otherwise she would have thought that she got away with something, just like the old days. But she has been really hard to deal with, now that she is home.

I finished my six weeks of parent education before the discharge, and that has really helped me. A few days after my daughter came home, she stole my car. I swore out a warrant for her arrest, something I learned how to do in the group. Now she is on the waiting list for a hearing in drug court, something else that is new for us. I will just keep applying the court consequences until I can get the leverage to get her back into a treatment program.

Once parents start receiving help for themselves, and they have taken advantage of this help, they are no longer as intimidated or paralyzed by their non-cooperative children. Regardless of how their adolescents are doing, these parents are getting well.

Dealing with outside enablers

It is always a relief to parents when their adolescents continue to make progress and are not discharged prematurely. As their teenagers grow and test their limits, some parents may have to address the outside enablers such as relatives and their teenager's school when they are making continued progress difficult. As parents get stronger, they are ready for this new challenge.

This father illustrates how far parents can go to support change in their schools:

We have become much more aware of the importance of natural consequences and that our son needs to be held accountable. He is in outpatient now, and a few weeks ago he and a few other people were caught using marijuana on school property. There were no school consequences, and I was furious.

I went to the principal. He was really upset that I was so angry. I told him that at least I didn't go to the police or the newspapers to talk about how the school is supporting illegal behavior and hurting kids. He said that they don't act because they have so many parents who are lawyers who threaten lawsuits when their kids get into trouble. He also said it isn't every kid who uses drugs, and it would give the wrong impression to the community if they talked about using at the high school.

I was really fed up and I even went to the superintendent. He was sympathetic, but that's it.

Schools don't want bad publicity, and they allow parents to scare them. I told the principal that they should call the police when kids do this kind of stuff. His mouth dropped. He said that I was the first parent that had said that. Lots of kids don't get help because they get bailed out. No wonder we have a teenage drug problem in our country.

I was really amazed that I took these steps. I have really learned a lot by being in our son's family treatment.

Many schools are doing an exceptional job in holding adolescents accountable for their behaviors. When schools do not follow through, however, parents may need to take action in order for changes to occur.

Taking care of yourself

Parents in treatment will continue to benefit from support at Families Anonymous, Nar-Anon, or Al-Anon meetings. As the treatment process continues, there will be many painful feelings to address, which will be discussed in the next three chapters. The road ahead will be both painful and rewarding. Recovery for adolescents and parents is the result of effort. Those who practice a strong program say that the effort is worth it. Parents are encouraged to keep going and to not give up.

CHAPTER 5

Working on Your Feelings

*"It doesn't happen all at once," said the Skin
Horse. "You become."*

—Margery Williams
The Velveteen Rabbit

WATCHING SOMEONE who is harmfully involved with drugs or alcohol is painful and lonely for those who are connected to that person as friends or family. In addition, your moods can change in an instant when your loved one is
doing well or if they are angry or if they come home intoxicated or high. It is
normal to feel that you are on a roller coaster that hurls you up or down as
you gasp for air. Sometimes it even feels like that roller coaster is broken,
and the speed is beyond the control of the operator. You are terrified as you
race forward, anticipating the crash.

This chapter will discuss the common feelings experienced by parents when
their teenagers are abusing drugs, how these feelings may be complicated by
their own painful childhood, and how to begin to reduce emotional pain
and isolation.

Common reactions

Your moods can fluctuate rapidly during the time when you are living with
the pain, isolation, and uncertainty of your adolescent's alcohol or drug
abuse. These parents' stories illustrate how extreme feelings affected them:

> *The most difficult part as a father was coming home each day and
> not knowing what I was facing. As I walked from the rapid transit stop,
> my chest would tighten and all the positive accomplishments of my day at
> the office would be forgotten. I was so filled with dread that I wanted to
> walk by the house. I knew the dive was coming in my personal roller
> coaster, and I didn't want to go down.*

* * * * *

[As a mom,] I created my own roller coaster. It all depended on how much I looked the other way. I spent a good part of my energy trying not to see what was going on. When it became too hard to deny, I really fell apart. All that was tied into living with alcoholics in my childhood—when we survived by denying—but I carried it right forward to how I dealt with my kids who were abusing drugs.

* * * * *

[As a dad,] I would go to work and it would be a safe haven, but then I would get a phone call that my son didn't show up at school or the police had picked him up somewhere. I made it through the day, but I made myself so ill that the next day I called in sick.

* * * * *

No matter what my wife and I did, nothing was working. We had done well as a family up to that time, and now everything was falling apart. As a father, my self-esteem went up and down and depended on how effective I felt that I could be. I had a lot of mood swings.

Stress in life is constant. A driver behind you tailgates; a work deadline looms; the line at the supermarket checkout puts a hold on your busy schedule. Every person's style of dealing with stress varies tremendously, however. You might habitually respond with anger when faced with stress or a situation that you can't control. You might respond by clenching your jaw, shouting at someone, driving more quickly, slamming your hand on a table, or inwardly roiling and taking antacids. Or your habitual response might be to feel overwhelmed in the face of stress. You might bury your head in your hands, sigh deeply, or dissolve into tears.

Having drug-abusing or drug-dependent adolescents challenges even the healthiest parents in terms of skills they otherwise use to cope with pain and frustration. It is normal to feel angry when teenagers are doing things that have legal or monetary consequences. It is also normal to feel frustrated when you get calls from the school or the police that your teenagers are truant or shoplifting or caught with alcohol on their breath. Parents often feel overwhelmed and resentful when a judge or relative chastises them for not controlling their teenagers. These outsiders do not appreciate the parents' sleepless nights when their teenagers were out beyond their curfew, the times they sat at home because their teenagers were grounded, or the arguments when parents told them not to leave the house. Parents who have faced these situations relate their frustrations with judgments:

> As a mother, the only thing I could have done further to control my son was to sit on him 24 hours a day like a fat crow sitting on an egg.

· · · · ·

> Nobody in the neighborhood actually came to the door to tell me I was a bad mother because my daughter was so out of control. But that's what I imagined that people were thinking. One time I got flip with a woman who asked about the beer bottles on the lawn. I told her something like, "If you have a problem with that, move."

There is usually a deep well of unexpressed pain beneath the justified defiance that results from an outsider's judgments. The mother of an addict describes the pain that lurks behind the isolation of many parents:

> My parents are blaming me for all the trouble my son is having. They don't understand how hard I have tried to keep him out of trouble.

The pain of being blamed for something you did not cause and did not want is severe. Many parents with a drug-abusing or drug-dependent teenager experience these feelings. The mother continues:

> The worst thing is that my parents blame me for bringing my drug-dealing son to a treatment program. They say, "If you had only been a better mother, he never would have gotten involved with drugs. He just needs a loving home."
>
> How can my own parents do this to me? I'm their daughter.

This story is very familiar. Family rejection is a cruel blow to a parent who is already feeling defeated. In this woman's example, a therapist who worked with her describes the family situation:

> Her husband had abandoned the young mother years before to raise this child alone, and she had worked two jobs to support them. I knew that she had tried many things to keep her son from continuing his destructive lifestyle, but none of them had worked. And now she was looking at the aftermath of what to many feels like a plane crash where they leave the rubble in a daze. She had no one to welcome her, no one to cheer her survival skills, no one to give her a hug.

Yes, parents with drug-abusing children are certainly challenged during this difficult time. It is important to understand how you deal with feelings of pain, loneliness, frustration, and stress as you reflect on your own personal roller coaster ride. You need to look at the choices you made in the past. You need to decide if you want to keep those choices or sweep them away. A father looking back reflects on how he needed help:

> I was an emotional wreck when we brought our 17-year-old son to treatment. I really needed help to stop how I was letting my life fall apart.

Dealing with feelings

All of us have a way to deal with feelings, a way we react.

The first step in evaluating your unique style that is to understand that you were born with some of your style. Children are different, even as infants. If you have more than one child, you are probably well aware of this. One child may have been feisty, another docile. Similarly, you were also born with a temperament.

Another way you develop your style is by what you experience in the culture. For example, if you are a woman in the US culture, you are usually nurtured to be more emotional and expressive than a man. In general, women have an easier time having intimate connections with other women in the workplace, on the playground, or in the locker room. A therapist working with parents describes one of these opportunities for connection:

> I swim laps every day, and I am amazed at how even a women's locker room is like a support group. I listen to women sharing tears, anxieties, and feelings of loneliness while changing into tennis or workout clothes, and I marvel at what a wonderful gift it is to have such a supportive environment.

Men in our culture, on the other hand, do not receive this same cultural gift of being expected to share emotions. A men's locker room, for example, is quite a different place.

As Merle Fossum says in his book *Catching Fire: Men Coming Alive in Their Recovery*:

> The one thing expected of the stereotypical "good man" in our culture is a healthy strain of toughness and strength. We teach our young

boys to be little soldiers or little cowboys. We over-emphasize one good
side of masculinity and teach boys to be strong, to never give in, to be
number one.[1]

Another aspect of our own personal culture is the family within which we
were raised. For example, men may have had a father who did not express
vulnerable feelings. Based on this experience, they model from these fathers
that men don't cry and that they simply "handle things." A father describes
what it was like to raise his son with more openness about feelings:

> *When my wife and I were raising our children, there was a wonder-*
> *ful record and songbook called Free to Be You and Me that we played to*
> *encourage them to be open with their feelings. One of the songs was "It's*
> *All Right To Cry," sung by a tough football tackle, Rosie Greer. "It's all*
> *right to cry," he bellowed. "It might make you feel better."*
>
> *I thought it was going to be so liberating for my five-year-old son if*
> *he could feel that way. I wish that I had grown up with that message.*

A father who has been working on his feelings comments on what is
expected of men:

> *Men aren't supposed to cry. How come women get to do everything?*
> *Totally unfair!*

Of course, it isn't only men who may have been encouraged by their family
to supress emotions. Women may have also been raised to be strong and
tough and not to cry. What do you believe about crying? Having the release
of tears during this difficult time can be a gift. Your ability to cry may be
hard to come by. Your experiences growing up can make your journey more
challenging.

Some parents grow up in what they consider normal families, but feelings
were not expressed. A father relates that experience and how it affected him
when his son began to experience difficulty:

> *I never saw either of my parents express emotions like crying until I*
> *was 11 years old. I remember it then because it was my mother who*
> *cried, and I was shocked. It was over something like a flood we saw in this*
> *little town in Kansas. But I don't remember her crying after that. And I*
> *would have really been shocked if my father ever cried. Even today, cry-*
> *ing seems strange to me, and I'm in my fifties.*

When my son was getting into trouble, my response was to think that my wife and I should just hunker down and once he got out of his teen years it would all be over. Her crying really bothered me, and I judged her harshly for it. We had a big wall between us. When we went into treatment, I realized that I had a lot of pain and sorrow underneath my exterior. I had such little experience expressing myself in more vulnerable ways, however, so it was really hard for me.

Parents who grow up in homes in which there is alcoholism, addiction, or mental illness can have an even greater difficulty expressing a range of feelings. Three parents describe what happens in these homes:

When I was growing up, you weren't really allowed to identify what was real. The drunkenness, the lies... We couldn't even empathize with my brother who was getting the brunt of my father's anger. It's like we had to pretend that it wasn't happening, so we couldn't even comfort him when his back was covered with welts from the razor strap. None of us cried, because there was nothing to cry about. We lived in a fantasy. I erased all my painful feelings.

· · · · ·

I was resentful that I didn't have parents like other kids, but I couldn't talk about that to anyone because I never told what was happening. I felt ashamed of my parents, but I couldn't talk about that either. Then I realized that I didn't respect my parents, but that feeling made me feel guilty about myself because you're supposed to respect your parents. The end result is that I squeezed every feeling out and I had nothing left to feel. I couldn't even feel good about a good day.

· · · · ·

When I was growing up I couldn't really comment on anything that was going on. My parents were like emotional mine-sweepers. Any expression wasn't safe. Even if some of their behavior was funny, you couldn't laugh. They would use anything you did as an excuse to get mad. I became numb. That's the way I lived my life.

When children grow up in chaotic homes where painful feelings are not expressed, it is also common to not trust outsiders. This can carry over to how parents deal with their pain when their teenagers are out of control. A number of parents explain how being numb paralyzed them:

As a child, I never trusted that anyone could help. It was such a hopeless situation. I felt the same way when the principal said we needed to get help for my son. I couldn't react. I had no feelings at all.

· · · · ·

Growing up, it was too much to think about talking about it all. I was told not to tell, so it felt like my whole world would fall apart if I did. I didn't know how, but I knew that it would. That's why I didn't want to talk about what my son was doing. And I didn't feel anything about it either.

· · · · ·

If family secrets were not kept when I was growing up, it would be an end to life as I knew it. The unknown would probably be worse. I didn't really allow myself to have feelings about what was going on. What would have been the point of that?

I had the same pattern when people started asking what I felt when my son had problems. I denied there were problems. I had no feelings. Everything was fine.

· · · · ·

Even though I was an adult and not living with my parents, I still felt unacceptable. That was part of having secrets. When I was growing up, my parents said that no one should know the truth about what was going on in our family. I thought that meant that the secrets we had were bad. People wouldn't like me if they knew the truth. The real me was unacceptable.

When my daughter started to get in trouble, the only feeling I had was feeling ashamed of who I was. That's all. Nothing about any pain from what she was doing. I lived this way until I brought her to treatment and started getting help for myself.

· · · · ·

I didn't trust my own feelings. For years I put my hand over my mouth when I laughed. I felt that whatever might come out might be inappropriate. I kept myself very compressed. I really didn't know what I felt when my son started getting into trouble.

· · · · ·

> *I was so numbed out from my childhood that when my daughter ran away I couldn't even answer the phone. What if she had called about coming to get her? I was a mess. But I couldn't feel anything, so I didn't even care if she called. I was numb.*

Many parents had a difficult time growing up. Many learned to turn off their feelings. This can have severe consequences when their teenagers start to abuse drugs and alcohol.

When parents question the style they use to handle their feelings, they go through a process that one therapist refers to as "spring cleaning":

> *We all know what it is like to walk through a basement or attic that is filled with clutter. Why does the clutter remain? "Maybe we will need those old magazines someday." That's why! Some of the items are even covered with mildew or mold or water stains, and they will never be usable. It is easier to leave them in their place, however, than to go through the effort of cleaning them out. Besides, they are familiar remnants of the past. "We can't get rid of that!"*

> *Such is also the case with your old reactions to life events.*

As illustrated by the following parents, many who struggle with adolescents abusing drugs want to substitute honest feelings for what they have inherited from their past:

> *I felt sad about a lot of things when I was a little girl, but I never told anyone. When I got to be a teenager, I turned all that sadness into rebellion. I was into a lot of things I now regret. As an adult, I didn't really start to express my sadness in healthy ways until my son went into treatment. I realized that I wanted to get healthier, too. I wanted to learn how to take care of myself better. I didn't like having all those resentments. There was a lot of sadness underneath them. I wanted to talk about my real feelings. I had to learn how to do this in treatment.*

· · · · ·

> *My brother and I were probably like most men. We didn't really talk about being sad when we were growing up although I know that we were. And my father didn't express those kinds of feeling either. We used action as a way to turn things around. When our son was so out of control, my actions didn't bring about change so my best way of dealing with things*

wasn't working. The problem was that I was sad and lonely and felt very inadequate, but I didn't really have any experience in talking about those kinds of feelings.

Complications from childhood

Parents who have grown up in families where there was a lot of pain have a special challenge while examining how they react to pain in the here and now. It is tough to survive complications such as watching abuse, being abused, suffering from emotional neglect, living with the mental illness of a parent, or dealing with parental alcoholism. Parents need to congratulate themselves on their survival skills and their strength. It has taken a special kind of courage to get through these difficult times. Parents do not have to be destroyed by these difficulties—they are even stronger for them.

On the other hand, parents need to look at how they survived and whether or not those survival skills are complicating their lives in the present. Two parents who sought help for their teens and themselves discuss how their children's substance abuse forced them to confront their own emotional issues:

> *My own personal work on my childhood began when my son started all his problems with drugs and alcohol. When I was a little girl, I would blame myself when my mother went on a binge. I would think that it wouldn't have happened if I had cleaned my room better or if I had found a better place to hide her gin bottles. I blamed myself in crazy ways like that with my own kid. I was so stuck in my old patterns that I didn't really see how out of control my son was. I totally let him off the hook. It was my fault, and it would all change if I got better. Thank God we brought him to treatment! It wasn't all about me. He was the one who was using. But I sure did need to work on myself, too.*

· · · · ·

> *The way I survived as a little girl turned into a nightmare when I saw my kids acting in the same ways I did. I had lived with rationalizations and denial, and now they were using them in terms of their own drug use. It was a nightmare because they learned that from me. It was really the incentive for me to get well. I was horrified.*

Parents who have this type of baggage from growing up an alcoholic home need to see that they are raising their teenagers with their childhood fears and anxieties. Many parents have a lot of clutter to sweep out in order to empower themselves as adults.

Understanding the ways that you got through difficult times helps you have respect and admiration for yourself. On the other hand, carrying the same survival skills to the present can add a special burden. These skills may have worked to get you to where you are today, but they were the survival skills of a child who depended on his parent for basic needs and emotional support. If your parents could not meet your needs as a child because of their own ill-nesses, you—like all children in such a situation—would have often used ways to deal with your feelings that are not healthy when you are grown up. Your own personal roller coaster ride during this time is even more terrify-ing if you use broken old reactions from childhood.

Complications in the here and now

Parents must work to understand and clean out the broken old reactions, because they have enough to deal with in the here and now. Having chil-dren who are abusing drugs and/or alcohol causes parents to go through a private hell. It is normal to experience pain as you live with your difficult sit-uation. It is normal to feel hurt, angry, afraid, guilty, resentful, and ashamed. As time goes on, and there is no change in your child's behavior, or it is worse, it is easy to feel hopeless, indifferent, and numb.

The box around the inside feelings in Figure 5-1 represents how people cut themselves off with defenses that are commonly used to deal with their inside pain. The defenses on the outside are common choices, often called rules, which family members operate under when they have a drug/alcohol abuser in the family.

When substance abuse occurs, it is common that family members do not want to talk about what is going on with outsiders or even with each other. For example, in the film and novel *The Prince of Tides*, the main character was tortured by horrifying past events that everyone in his family had observed but no one talked about, even while they were happening. The mother of a 17-year-old, drug-abusing son who entered treatment describes how the silence worked in her family:

> *When I was a child and living with my two younger brothers and baby sister, my stepfather was drunk a few days after Christmas, and he*

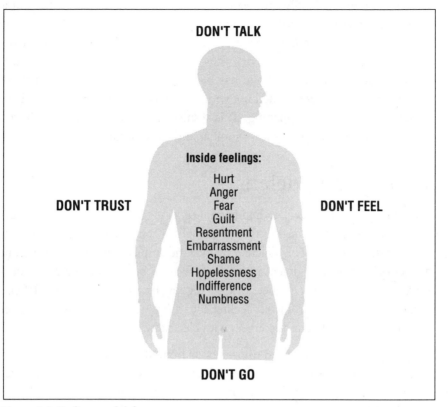

DON'T TALK

Inside feelings:

Hurt
Anger
Fear
Guilt
Resentment
Embarrassment
Shame
Hopelessness
Indifference
Numbness

DON'T TRUST

DON'T FEEL

DON'T GO

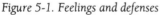

Figure 5-1. Feelings and defenses

*put our tree in the blazing fireplace because he didn't want to carry it out
to the curb. My mother was drunk, too, so she wasn't really in a condition to stop him. Us kids were all in the living room and saw him do it,
but I don't remember that anyone said anything. I do recall that the tree
seemed to blow up, and the part sticking out on the floor ignited the rugs.
When the fire trucks came, my brothers and I just stood across the street
and watched the house burn. I held my sister, and I remember that she
was screaming.*

*I don't remember that my brothers and I talked about it at the time.
There were a lot of things like that happening that were scary, but we sort
of got used to them. We didn't even react to things as time went on.*

*When we were adults, I asked my two brothers if they remembered
the fire. It was hard to talk about it even then.*

Isolation within the family can result in having difficulty asking for help. It is also common to not trust that anyone can help you. This often leads to lying about what is going on. We are not sure of what others will do with the information, and we even fear that they will somehow hold us responsible. After all, our addict or alcoholic has blamed us. We have come to believe that we must have done something wrong. Otherwise this out-of-control situation would not be happening. This results in a type of loyalty to even a bad situation because it is at least familiar and the unknown could be worse.

Feelings and defenses

A defense mechanism is a normal mental process that we use to protect ourselves from something in life that is thought to be unpleasant, uncomfortable, or threatening. The defense blocks the unpleasant matter from our awareness. By using a defense, we think we feel better, but we block ourselves from the true experience of what is going on inside of us. The defense makes us disconnect from our feeling like a broken toaster that no longer functions because it cannot connect with electricity.

Defense mechanisms are used to protect us from life traumas that might otherwise overwhelm us. For those who had painful childhoods, the defenses helped them survive. In the here and now, parents report that the defenses they used to survive out-of-control children helped them get through the stress. But the personal cost to them was high.

As already expressed by several parents, hopelessness, indifference, and numbness mean that you do not let yourself feel anything at all. This can be dangerous. As psychotherapist Belleruth Naperstek writes in *Your Sixth Sense*:

> *It may initially seem kinder to protect ourselves by closing our hearts down and cutting ourselves off from our feelings, [but] it doesn't really work that way, at least not in the long run. The exhaustion of burnout actually comes from being shut down and disconnected from the vast energy supply that our feelings generate.*[2]

The lyrics of the Simon and Garfunkel song "I Am a Rock" can describe the emotional experience parents often have when their teenagers are abusing drugs and alcohol. These powerful images describe turning oneself into a rock as a way to cope with pain. Loneliness intensifies behind a fortress of walls that could be compared to the defenses parents use to shield themselves from this pain. The song ends with the reason for this isolation:

> And a rock feels no pain
>
> And an island never cries.[3]

A therapist who uses the song "I Am a Rock" when working with parents describes what happens:

> When I play this song in my parent group, I usually watch tears slide down the cheeks of both men and women as they shift in their seats, afraid of watchful eyes. They recognize themselves in the words, and they are afraid.

The mother of a drug-dependent 17-year-old relates to the image of a fortress of walls:

> When my son was getting into so much trouble, my only life away from work was surfing the Internet. I was hiding in the room where we had our computer. I had no life.

The father of an addict looks back at his experience and relates to closing himself off from those who were there to help him:

> Friends of mine would call to ask me to play golf or tennis, and I told them I was busy. My excuses worked at the beginning, but after a while we all knew I was lying. My friends had to move on. They told me later how arrogant I was and how I pushed people away. That was such an irony because I really needed friends.

Two parents describe similar ways they cut off support during the time when their teens were abusing drugs:

> I just threw myself into extra projects at work. I stopped eating because I was too busy. It was insane. I was like this little island unto myself.

· · · · ·

> I was determined that I wouldn't let my daughter's problems get to me, so I decided to be tough and not let myself feel anything. And I didn't want to be close to my friends because maybe they would start me crying. I didn't even let myself watch movies, and I looked away at those

commercials for Mother's Day. I was not going to let my feelings get to me. I told myself that I could handle this, and no one was able to help anyway.

A therapist who works with parents describes a family situation that also speaks to the isolation felt by parents whose adolescents are abusing drugs:

A hefty father who worked in the steel mills told me a story that I have not forgotten. He confessed that he had spent a recent day hiding in his house while his wife was at work and his daughter was in elementary school. He was numbing himself with daytime television while his hand-cuffed son pounded against a locked basement door.

The handcuffs had been applied the previous evening after his son terrorized the family in a drunken rage, smashing furniture and a glass vase collection belonging to his mother. Afterward, the stocky 17-year-old had collapsed in the basement on an old couch. His mother and sister had barricaded themselves with a dresser behind a locked bedroom door, and his father had handcuffed him while he slept. When the son woke the next morning, the basement door was locked.

"Did you think about calling the police?" I asked.

"No. What would they think of me that I couldn't even control my own kid?"

Unfortunately, this story is familiar to many parents. Many are, indeed, prisoners in their own homes during this difficult period when their teenagers are abusing drugs. The roller coaster ride for many parents is terrifying. It is normal for many parents to close off their feelings, to numb themselves, to be a rock. Chapter 7, *Communication and Relationships*, will elaborate on costs parents see for themselves and their teenagers by not working on their feelings.

Taking care of yourself

Examining the choices you make to deal with pain is a very demanding process. You may also feel defensive because you do not want to focus on your feelings. Parents often feel that staying with their pain would only paralyze them. It would only make things worse.

On the other hand, many parents who are further along in the process of examining themselves say that the pain is there, and they contribute to their own burnout by stuffing it and not sharing it. Parents also relate that they suffer from colds, lower back pain, or insomnia. Some parents take drugs, drink alcohol, or overeat to deal with their isolation and loneliness. In addition, they report that because they stuff their feelings, they know they are not good decision-makers when it comes to what to do about their drug/alcohol-abusing teenager. They want to be in touch with what they really feel because they know that decisions will then be easier.

Parents who want to be healthier, and who want to improve as decision-makers, know they need to examine their own feelings and how they express them. They know they need to think carefully about the choices they are making with their feelings.

Self-examination can be painful. Special care needs to be taken to continue this difficult process. Many parents have forgotten how to take care of themselves because they have been so focused on their teenagers. Nurturing yourself can make it easier to deal with what is going on, however, and helps you stick with the changes you are making. Examples of nurturing yourself might include buying a single rose or a bouquet for your desk or nightstand. You might remember that you used to like a soothing herbal bath or talking with a friend you have not spoken with for a long time. If you have escaped into workaholic habits, you can take time for a walk or call a friend to play golf or tennis.

At this time of intense examination, parents have often found relief in hobbies they abandoned months or even years ago. One mother went home from a session at a treatment program to create a stained glass hanging as a present for her therapist. The mother spoke of it with pride, tears streaming down her face:

> I started it when I got home from that feeling session. It was time to start caring about myself. I plan to continue with my stained glass as a hobby and to exhibit a collection of my art in a craft show.

What can you do to start caring for yourself at this difficult time? Taking care of yourself will benefit your entire family as well as take you off your roller coaster. Remember, you're worth it!

Some specific suggestions:

- As you deal with painful feelings, it is very important to connect with supportive friends and family members. Many parents will also have a religious congregation where supportive people can be found to help with feelings of pain and suffering. Parents who do not have this spiritual type of support available are encouraged to seek it out to see if it helps.

- If there are painful feelings left over from childhood, it may be helpful to seek a therapist. There are many therapists who are trained to help people talk about these feelings. Therapists can help you work through this pain and the effect it is having on you today.

- Find an Al-Anon, Nar-Anon, or Families Anonymous meeting in your area if you have not already started to attend. You will receive a great deal of support during this difficult period when your teenager is abusing drugs or alcohol or has started an assessment or treatment. You will also find helpful material about feelings on the literature table at these meetings.

- For those who grew up in an alcoholic home and are trying to connect with their painful childhood, it might also be helpful to attend Adult Children of Alcoholics meetings. These are listed in Al-Anon meeting schedules or through calling your local Al-Anon Central Office, which is listed in your phone book.

- Viewing films in the privacy of your home is an excellent way to get in touch with feelings from your past that you have buried with layers and layers of defenses. Appendix A, *Resources*, lists some films recommended for looking at childhood issues such as growing up in an alcoholic or abusive home, or growing up with a mentally ill parent.

- Seek out recordings that have emotion. A wide range of music brings out emotions—classical, popular, world music, or recordings of nature. Dust off your old recordings. A selection of music that has been helpful to other parents going through this process is listed in Appendix A.

- Suggestions for reading about issues discussed in this chapter are also listed in Appendix A.

CHAPTER 6

Harmful Consequences from Normal Feelings

*What appears to be the end may really be a
new beginning.*

—Anonymous

As PARENTS CONTINUE to examine ways they deal with the painful feelings of parenting substance-abusing adolescents, they understand in even greater depth the importance of this personal evaluation. They realize that their pain, loneliness, and despair are not going away. They know that whatever they are trying to do to help their teenagers is not working. These parents understand that they need to somehow change their situation. If they do not, things will only get worse.

This chapter will discuss how parents' normal, painful feelings can interfere with their ability to help themselves as well as their drug-abusing teenagers. It will conclude with a discussion of ways that parents can begin to change patterns that have only made the situation worse.

Consequences and codependency

Parents can perpetuate their pain, loneliness, despair, and hopelessness when they are codependent with their drug-abusing teenagers. Codependency is a word that is often used to describe the common patterns of interaction that exist between drug and alcohol abusers/dependents and their families. It is used sometimes glibly in our culture or by the media, sometimes incorrectly. Being codependent means that you are so interconnected with the feelings and behaviors of another person that the boundaries between you are nearly indistinguishable. If they are depressed, you are depressed. If they are happy, you are happy. If they are succeeding in life,

119

you are also succeeding. However you are doing or feeling is in direct reaction to the people around you. You are enmeshed with them. Who you are depends on who they are. It is almost as if you are a yo-yo dangling on their string, totally at the mercy of what they decide to do or feel. You have lost your own identity.

Codependent living patterns are dangerous and destructive and rob us of the energy we need to lead productive lives. These patterns can cause pain to parents and teenagers and stand in the way of getting help. A simple physical exercise illustrates the pain that codependence can bring. Lace the fingers of your hands together. This interlacing is an image of how codependency works. Now push your fingers hard against each other and you experience pain in between each finger. Push them harder and harder, and you are really in pain. Codependency gets worse if you do not address it in earlier stages, and it keeps getting more intense. Chapter 7, *Communication and Relationships*, discusses codependent interactions in more depth. This chapter focuses on the damage from the feelings that occur when parents are codependent.

Authors such as Melody Beattie, in her books *Codependent No More* and *Beyond Codependency*, and Sharon Wegscheider-Cruse, in her book *Another Chance: Hope and Health for the Alcoholic Family*, describe the natural process whereby family members are impacted by a drug/alcohol abuser. According to Wegscheider-Cruse:

> *In the interests of their own personal survival, the members of the family assume behavior patterns that will maintain a balance in the [family] system. In time they will [all] follow the same long, slow path to personal disintegration, both individually and as a family.*[1]

Patterns of feelings

If there are drug-abusing teenagers in families and that problem is not being addressed, the family members, including the parents, will become more and more dysfunctional. The substance abusers' self-worth will continue to disintegrate as they continue their use and their harmful consequences. Their poor self-esteem will be expressed in negative ways, such as striking out at parents, brothers, and sisters. By this time, as their substance abuse progresses, they will lose touch with their true, vulnerable feelings. They substitute those true feelings with false emotions that are less painful.

Table 6-1 illustrates what is happening to the substance-abusing adolescent and to the family members.

Table 6-1. Feelings and Behaviors in Substance-Abusing Families

Abuser's True Feelings	Abuser's Behavior	Family Members' Feelings
Guilt, self-hatred	Self-righteous, blaming	Guilt, self-hatred
Fear	Aggressive, angry	Fear
Helplessness	Controlling (of others)	Helplessness
Hurt	Abusive	Hurt
Loneliness	Rejecting, grandiose	Loneliness
Low self-worth	Judging, criticizing	Low self-worth

Many parents relate to the feelings described in Table 6-1. These stories illustrate the normal feelings of guilt, self-hatred, fear, helplessness, hurt, loneliness, and worthlessness that parents struggle with when their child is abusing drugs:

I was so depressed when our 17-year-old son went to treatment, because I had really tried hard to be a good mother. My own childhood was a mess, and I was determined to not be like my own parents. My husband was a great father, too. We really felt like we had failed. It was our fault.

· · · · ·

I felt absolutely worthless as a mother when my son had so much trouble. I was sinking in muck, in quicksand. There was no action I could take. I tried checking his homework to make sure that he did it, I tried sitting by the door so he wouldn't leave, and I tried hanging up when his friends called. I even drove to school to pick him up when classes were over.

But he wouldn't do his homework, and he would leave out a window, and it didn't matter that I hung up on his friends. And when I went to get him at school, he wasn't there. I didn't feel that I could ask friends to help because then they would know how bad it was. They had nice kids. If the truth was out, it would just close off opportunities for my son to be with nice kids. Besides, I didn't want my friends to know that I was a bad mother.

One night I just started to cry when I thought about this massage therapist I was paying 50 dollars a week just so I could feel someone touch me. The only way I could get close to someone was to pay her.

• • • • •

This was such a difficult time as a father because our son's behavior changed so dramatically. We had no understanding of what was causing it, and we had no idea of what to do about it. I felt totally helpless as a father. It challenged my basic confidence in myself.

• • • • •

I was upset as a mother that our daughter had forgotten all the values we had taught her. And then I questioned myself. Maybe we hadn't done enough. I started to feel guilty that I wasn't a good enough parent.

• • • • •

My own self-esteem as a father really went down because there was such a change in our son. I couldn't understand how this could have happened. Professionally I have to travel abroad to unfamiliar places where I don't necessarily know the language. That's what this felt like: I was a stranger in my own home. It's like I had traveled to a foreign place, and I had no sense of connection to the area. I didn't know how to talk to my son. I didn't know who he was.

• • • • •

My son is a lot bigger than I am. Even his father was afraid of him. He was only 16 before he entered treatment, so he was a child, and we were the adults. Our fear was so strong, however, that we treated him like the parent.

• • • • •

When my husband went out of town, I was terrified that my daughter would do something to hurt me. She definitely got her way with whatever she wanted to do because of this. She used her anger and her size to intimidate.

• • • • •

I don't think that my husband and I denied what was going on, but we were too tired to intervene. The feeling of helplessness was overwhelming. Our daughter was out of control. I was the stay-at-home mother and I was really worn out by trying to change something.

• • • • •

The lowest point for me as a mother was when I found out about all the lies my son had told. How could he have done this? I felt really hurt because we had tried hard to give him values. How could he let us down? I say this now and realize how far I have come in understanding his addiction. But I took it all personally at the beginning.

• • • • •

As a mother, I had so many problems with my mood swings that my boss told me that I needed to go to a counselor if I was going to keep my job. We had this kind of help right there at work, so it was easy for me. But I'm a professional. People pay me to solve big problems. Getting help because I couldn't control my daughter was humiliating. I wondered who knew about it. I was sure that people were talking about me behind my back.

Physical reactions

In the days before managed care, there were many 30-day treatment programs at places like Sierra Tucson in Arizona or Lutheran Deaconess in Minneapolis where adolescent treatment specialists would refer severely codependent parents. This extended inpatient treatment was necessary because these parents were debilitated by their painful feelings and had harmful consequences such as compulsions, stress disorders, relationship addictions, severe depression, eating or food disorders, and their own chemical abuse. Insurance-reimbursed treatment was done in the context of how family members become enmeshed, or codependent, with a suffering relative.

Unfortunately, due to restrictions under managed care, these 30-day specialized programs that were totally covered by insurance no longer exist. They provided a much needed service, and more people were able to access them because of this reimbursement. Sierra Tucson still offers a 30-day residential program, but only four to five days, at best, will be covered. Codependency problems are also treated in psychiatric wards, outpatient counseling, or in a few week-long outpatient programs that are often called workshops. Some of these programs are listed in Appendix A, *Resources*.

Enlightened medical internists, such as gastroenterologist Gary Gottlieb, MD, of Cleveland, know that the stress for parents as they deal with a child's out-of-control behavior can have serious medical consequences. Dr. Gottlieb addresses this in his Mind/Body Institute where he and his associates offer month-long workshops and support groups on mind/body medicine. According to Dr. Gottlieb:

> Mind/body medicine is a system of healing based on the concept that the mind and body are one, not separated. In my medical practice, I have found time and time again that patients with chronic complaints are undergoing emotional stress that they are not handling very well. If I am going to successfully treat their physical problems, I have to also teach them how to handle their stress.

Physicians, therapists, and others across the United States and Canada who support this holistic approach believe in the need to show their patients that the way they respond to situations in their everyday lives may be affecting their health. At the Mind/Body Institute, Dr. Gottlieb and his associates conduct interactive lectures, discussions, and small group exercises that are designed to help patients respond to everyday situations more effectively. Individuals meet together for two hours every week for six weeks, and there are also home reading and practice assignments. According to Dr. Gottlieb, those who have participated in programs like this have very positive things to say about the results:

> I see people understanding how physical symptoms and moods are related to certain events in their lives. They are learning that they have a choice about what they do with their feelings. For example, they see how to shift their mood when they wake up at night so they can more easily get back to sleep. They learn how to deal with what is making it impossible for them to function. This saves them from all the physical symptoms that are a result of not knowing how to make better choices.

Parents under severe stress from their children's drug/alcohol abuse can relate to the mind/body connections described by Dr. Gottlieb:

> I was a physical wreck as a mother when we went through our teenager's drug abuse. I had so many of those calling-in-sick days from feeling so ill that my supervisor confronted me. He said that I was doing a great job when I was there. But the operative word was "there," and it wasn't very often. He made it very clear that my job was on the line if I didn't get help. He even drove me to a Mood Disorder Clinic at a local hospital so I could sign up. I was going to get fired if I didn't attend, so I went to treatment for seven days straight. It changed my life.

As a father, I kept all my feelings inside about my kid stealing and the police officer coming. There were days when I felt that I couldn't keep my eyes open because I didn't want to see what was in front of me. I almost drove into trees several times. It's a miracle that I didn't kill myself.

Two mothers who had treatment for mind/body connections describe how treatment helped:

When my son was so heavily into drugs, I had diarrhea and gas from loading up on sugar and carbohydrates, and I felt parched and dry all the time because I stopped drinking water. I didn't even have the sensation of being hungry. Then I would binge on sugar, junk stuff like Twisters. I would stuff myself when I was alone in the kitchen or when I was watching the dryer in the laundry room. At some level, I knew I was out of control, and I didn't want anyone to see me. But I also wanted to deny it to myself, just like I wanted to deny what my son was doing.

· · · · ·

My doctor gave me an antidepressant, but he also said that I needed to go to treatment to talk about my feelings. When I did that, my stomachaches and headaches stopped. My daughter was still running away and calling me a bitch, but I was getting healthier in how I dealt with it.

Physical reactions to emotional pain are common in families where there is drug abuse. These parents show that if intervention does not occur, there can be catastrophic results.

Codependency, enabling, and parenting traps

There are harmful consequences to drug/alcohol abusing teenagers when parents are feeling emotionally numb and physically burnt-out, or—at the other extreme—when parents are so consumed with anger that their loved ones worry about them getting an ulcer or having a heart attack. All of these emotions usually lead to enabling.

"Enabling" is actually a very nice word that means helping. We use the word to indicate when someone's efforts help us to achieve a goal. Your supervisor's support, for example, could enable a raise from the president of your company. When talking about substance abuse, however, enabling is not a nice word unless you are the person who is abusing the mood-altering substance. In fact, abusers *love* the person who enables. Why? This is the person who is going to help them toward their goal of continuing their drug and/or alcohol abuse. Of course they love the enabler!

Enabling actions are those that take away the harmful consequences of drug/ alcohol abusers' behavior. Enabling might mean lying to cover up that your adolescents are staying home sick due to a binge or calling them in sick to school when they have actually run away and a report should be filed on them at the police station.

Enabling is also doing your teenagers' chores when they refuse to do them themselves. Enabling is when parents find drug paraphernalia or drugs in their homes and do not file possession charges or make an appointment for an assessment. Enabling is when parents deny, rationalize, or minimize what is going on. Because of this, parents help drug abusers deny, rationalize, and minimize their drug and alcohol use and the consequences from that use.

Parents who have been in treatment relate how enabling worked when their adolescents were abusing alcohol and drugs. The following stories show the many dimensions of enabling:

> As a mom, I had so many excuses for my daughter if she was abus-ing drugs. If she hadn't thought of one, it was almost as if I was saying, "Here, take this excuse!"

· · · · ·

> My biggest problem as a mom was agreeing with my son that he wouldn't have gotten drunk and trashed the basement if his father had been nicer to him that afternoon. We were divorced, and I hated the guy, so it was okay with me to blame all my son's problems on him.
>
> I really dismissed all of my son's misbehavior. I looked the other way.

· · · · ·

> My wife was really on a witch-hunt where my daughter was con-cerned. My daughter could do nothing right. She would tell me what a good father I was, so I had an agreement with her to not tell her mother when she came home late or left the house when she was grounded.

· · · · ·

As a mom, I felt that our school system never addressed my daughter's problems. When she got in trouble for having alcohol on her breath, I yelled at the principal when he called me on the phone. My daughter said that she never would have gotten into trouble if she had a decent education there. Of course, it never occurred to me that smelling like gin at nine in the morning is not normal.

Three fathers relate to how they also looked the other way and engaged in enabling:

We had this red Karmann Ghia convertible, and my son always seemed to get in trouble when he was in that car. I talked a friend into keeping it at his house. I was sure that things would get better. Then he got into trouble in my Honda. It took a while for me to realize that it wasn't the car's fault.

· · · · ·

I blamed all my daughter's problems on her friends. But she chose those friends. I didn't want to look at her part in all this.

· · · · ·

I blamed my son's problems on the neighborhood we lived in. It was the whole town, actually. We decided to move to this suburb where it seemed safe. The new house was expensive, but it didn't matter. We would do anything for our kids. Then my son started to hang out with the same kind of kids there. It was sad because we really liked our old neighbors. We had moved for nothing.

Many parents talk about the family conflicts and the guilt that would result in letting their kids off the hook:

My wife and I would fight about what to do about our daughter while she was standing there complaining that we didn't trust her. Of course we had no reason to trust her, but she always had a way of getting us to be so mad at each other that we stopped paying attention to her. She would just walk out the door and go and party somewhere. Then she used the excuse that we were fighting, and she had to get out of the house. We felt guilty, so we thought it probably was a good excuse. She told me later that she would try to get us to fight. It let her off the hook.

• • • • •

I felt guilty about divorcing my husband, so I would give my son any-thing he wanted. I understand that he used me. Actually, he told me this himself when he started to get well.

• • • • •

My son's father is in prison, so I felt sorry for him. It's like I had to give him the love of two parents. My son told me in treatment that he took advantage of this when he was in trouble. I didn't want him to suffer any more, so I thought that the consequences were too hard when other people recommended them. It's lucky that the court finally put him in jail. The way things were going, he would have died because I looked the other way.

• • • • •

My husband is a successful attorney, and he isn't home much. I felt sorry for my son and tried to make it up to him when his dad was hard on him for getting into trouble. In my own mind, I thought it was because his father was gone. That's why he got into trouble.

It never occurred to me that our son might be an addict, and it didn't matter whether his dad was home or not. Even when the dads are home, kids can get in trouble with drugs.

• • • • •

We adopted our daughter, so we felt like we had to be extra-special parents. We made up so many excuses for her when she got into trouble.

• • • • •

As a loving father, I didn't want to believe that my sweet daughter was abusing drugs. Boy, did she manipulate this! One time a friend told me that I was in la-la land where she was concerned. I got mad at him, but he said he wanted me to see that movie Go Ask Alice. The girl looked a lot like my daughter. There was this one scene where she was stoned at this family picnic, and the parents couldn't see it. That was a turning point for me. I realized what a fool I was. Thank God my friend accepted my apology. He saved my daughter's life.

These parents illustrate the many excuses, rationalizations, and minimiza-tions that constitute enabling. What they said also illustrates how often enabling happens with good intentions that are manipulated by drug/alco-hol abusing children.

Enabling and codependency

Why do parents enable? Reasons relate to the basic human need to feel loved and appreciated or, the opposite, to not feel rejected. Also, parents choose to have or adopt children because they want to be parents. They feel it will be a pleasurable experience to have children. They see themselves as capable of the love that will be needed to raise them.

It is natural for parents to have lifelong desires to help their children. It is common to want to protect them, teach them, and spare them pain. Parents can all relate to the longing to be good, loving parents.

Unfortunately, in a desire to continue their drug and alcohol abuse, teenagers usually take advantage of their parents and manipulate their longings. As part of their love relationship with mood-altering chemicals, they use their well-meaning parents in any way possible so that they can continue abusing drugs and alcohol. This is why these basic parental needs or longings are called "parenting traps" when you have drug- or alcohol-abusing teenagers. Parents get trapped by these longings to be good and loving parents as if they were in quicksand. They go down in defeat, unable to help themselves or their adolescents. Their situations only get worse.

Addicts or alcoholics who are in the process of getting well recognize their old manipulations. These behaviors are used to help them continue their love relationship with drugs and alcohol. Teens who have been in treatment for addiction describe the manipulations that are common to adolescent alcoholics/addicts:

> I knew that my mom would back down if I got in her face. She was afraid of my anger, and I used that to get what I wanted.

· · · · ·

> My parents were divorced, and they hated each other. I could always get what I wanted by telling each of them that they were the best parent.

· · · · ·

> My mom really liked to go to my school and tell them off when I got into trouble. It seemed to make her feel good to try and solve my problems. I really liked it when she took over because no one paid attention to me.

· · · · ·

My dad really wanted me to stay in my private school. He had gone there and so had my grandfather. It was like a family prestige thing. When I was kicked out for drinking, he raised holy hell about it. He even said he would tell other people not to contribute. I thought it was pretty cool when he did that, but I was also embarrassed. The good thing is that the headmaster didn't back down. That's how I eventually got to treatment.

· · · · ·

My father had a terrible temper, and he would really get mad when I did something wrong. He would scare me sometimes, but I could beat him, and he knew it. One time I went after him when I was drunk, and a neighbor called the cops. They told my dad that he was the problem. They didn't even seem to care that I was wasted. I thought that was cool, and I threw it back in his face anytime he got upset when I came home drunk. He was scared of his anger. I used that to get what I wanted.

· · · · ·

One night I was out with my friends, and we got so drunk that we decided to knock over all the mailboxes on this long road in our town. When the cops started asking around, I lied about it to my parents. They knew I was out, and I think they even thought I was involved, but they told the cops I was at home watching TV with them. That was really funny because we never watched TV together. I was glad they lied, though. They didn't want to look bad in the community. I could get away with just about anything.

· · · · ·

My dad wanted to believe that I was this perfect little girl. For example, I would come home smelling of alcohol, but he told my mom that I didn't drink and they would fight about it. My mom was on to me, and I hated her. I told my dad he should get a divorce, and I would live with him. I could do no wrong in his eyes. It was such a joke. I used to laugh about him with my friends while we were getting high.

These manipulations need to be understood in the context of the substance abuse process where the alcohol/drug abuser's major preoccupation is with continuing their drug and alcohol use. However, the alcohol/drug abusers talking above had cooperation in this manipulation from their loving parents. When the parents' needs created an opening to be taken advantage of, the substance abusers used it to maximum advantage.

Parenting traps

The parents' desires to be good and loving can lead to the following parenting traps. Each trap is followed by a story from a parent or parents that illustrates the trap and what happens when parents fall in:

- **Trap number one.** Your struggles affect my serenity. My mental attention focuses on solving your problems or relieving your pain.

  I was trying to find a way to reach my daughter. She had so many talents. I was so afraid that she would die. My job as a parent was to prevent that from happening. I drove myself nuts trying to learn everything. I was trying to control that she would be okay.

  The trap for me was that I couldn't even think straight, because I had overwhelmed myself. My daughter took advantage of this. I was so confused and burned out from worry that I couldn't even hold her accountable to rules I had set. It was easier to let her do whatever she wanted.

  · · · · ·

  My feelings about myself had a lot to do with how my kids were doing. I took my parenting very seriously. When my daughter was failing, I was helpless. My own self-worth went down dramatically. This affected my confidence in everything I did, even when it wasn't directly related to parenting. I started doing poorly everywhere. I had no way at all to feel good about myself.

  The trap was that I had lost the ability to really help my daughter because I had no confidence in who I was. I lost my ability to concentrate and this affected my decision-making. My mental attention had been so focused on her that I burned myself out.

- **Trap number two.** My mental attention is focused on manipulating you to do it "my way."

  The trap for me was trying to cure my son's problem myself. If I learned enough, then I could fix it. I knew he was in a difficult situation, so I tried to interject myself in a more forceful way. His behaviors only got worse. Things became very volatile in the house when I started to yell a lot. I was out of control with my anger. The attention was more on me being the problem. My son used that to manipulate for what he wanted.

- **Trap number three.** My self-esteem is bolstered by relieving your pain.

    I fell right in the trap of feeling good because I was helping my daughter out of trouble. She used that to avoid consequences. She got worse, and I really regret that I was such an enabler.

- **Trap number four.** Your clothing and personal appearance is dictated by my desires. You are a reflection of me.

    My daughter dressed nicely and got decent grades, and I wanted to believe that she was like those kids in Seventeen magazine. People would even say that she looked like a model. Kids like her didn't have trouble with drugs. I wanted to believe that she was perfect.

    The trap for me is that I looked the other way. I wanted my own dreams.

· · · · ·

My lowest point when my son was using was when I had a rage attack and hit him after I saw him near a movie theatre looking stoned and dirty with all those rings on his face and his ears. I was with some friends. I was sure they were judging me that I had a son who looked like he did. When he came home later, I went after him. I am embarrassed now that I got so out of control.

The trap for me was that I thought if I could change the way my son looked, everything would improve. It was also an ego thing for me. I had my own image to protect. I was so focused on appearance that I lost perspective.

- **Trap number five.** Your behavior is dictated by my desires. You are a reflection of me.

    When I saw my son struggling, I couldn't acknowledge it. He wasn't like me so it was as if he didn't exist. He wasn't even there. When my wife talked about his behaviors, I tuned her out. I couldn't even respond and get him some help. She had to take over because I was so numb.

    This was a real trap for us because my wife didn't get support from me. This delayed our son getting help.

· · · · ·

The way I looked at my kids when they were using drugs was with blinders on. Their behaviors were according to my desires of how I wanted to see them. This is why I had so many rationalizations for what they did. My rationalizations trapped me into not getting help.

- **Trap number six.** My fear of rejection determines what I say or do.

    My daughter would tell me that I was a poor excuse for a mother or that if I really loved her I would give her money or do something else she wanted from me. I was so afraid of her rejection that I would give her anything. What a trap that was!

- **Trap number seven.** My fear of your anger determines what I say or do.

    Before my son came to treatment, there was one time when I found drugs he had hidden in his room. He heard me call the police to tell them to send an officer over because I was having trouble with my son. He came into the room with a baseball bat, his face red and his nostrils flaring like a bull. He told me to call the police station to tell them that everything was okay, or I would regret it. I was so afraid of him that I made the call.

    His anger controlled me to such an extent that I never thought that I could call the police later or look up the number for one of those abuse hotlines. My fear of his anger was my biggest trap.

- **Trap number eight.** I put my values aside to connect with you.

    I was not present in my emotional life when all this was happening. I couldn't take it any more. I even lied about things my kid did. I knew I was doing it, but at least my kid was nice to me when he found out that I stood up for him.

• • • • •

    I look back now and I am ashamed that I put my values aside to connect with him. My enabling was horrible.

    I didn't really realize that my kids had choices independent of me because I sort of bought that everything they did was a reflection of me and I must have failed if they did something wrong. If the police came over, I didn't want to file charges because it really wasn't my kid's fault, it was mine for not being a good enough parent. What a trap!

When I started getting help for myself, I realized that I didn't teach my son to lie and steal. He made those choices.

- **Trap number nine.** I value your opinion and way of doing things more than my own.

  When my 14-year-old daughter started disobeying home rules, she had all kinds of reasons for why she didn't need a curfew or why her jacket had the sweet smell of marijuana. My instincts told me she was lying, but I was losing confidence in myself because she was so persuasive. I started to value her opinion more than my own. I forgot that I was the parent and she was only 14.

- **Trap number ten.** The quality of my life is in relation to the quality of your life.

  I was so enmeshed with my son that whatever mood he was in, I was in. Whatever trouble he was in, I was totally focused on how to get him out of it. There was no quality to my life whatsoever. I had no life of my own. This was a big parenting trap. I was so enmeshed that I couldn't think straight about what my son was doing and how to hold him accountable.

It can be painful to read how these parents' self-esteem was so debilitated by their valiant attempts to help their teenagers. What a rotten deal! Yes, this is true. But, unfortunately, this is a common occurrence in families where there is a drug/alcohol abuser. This is why it is so important for parents to understand and evaluate the style they have when they are under stress, and to look at their codependency patterns.

When you think of your own personal roller coaster, it is possible to get off.

Parents have the option to respond in new ways to out-of-control adolescents. The following letters from a substance abuser and an enlightened parent are helpful in developing more effective attitudes and behaviors. The first is an anonymous letter circulated by Families Anonymous to help parents:

An open letter to my family,

I am a drug abuser. I need help.

Don't solve my problems for me. This only makes me lose respect for you and for myself.

Don't lecture, blame, moralize, scold, or argue whether I'm stoned or sober. It may make you feel better, but it only makes the situation worse.

Don't accept my promises. The nature of my illness prevents me from keeping them, even though I mean them at the time. Promises are only my way of postponing pain. And don't keep switching agreements; if an agreement is made, stick to it.

Don't lose your temper with me. It will destroy you and any possibility of helping me.

Don't let your anxiety for me make you do what I should do for myself.

Don't believe everything I tell you. Often I don't even know the truth—let alone tell it.

Don't try to cover up or spare me the consequences of my using. It may reduce the crisis, but it will make my illness worse.

Above all, don't run away from reality as I do. Drug dependence, my illness, gets worse as my using continues.

Start now to learn, to understand, to plan for recovery. Find Families Anonymous, whose groups exist to help families in just your situation.

I need help—from a doctor, a psychologist, a counselor, from some people in a self-help program who are recovering from a drug problem themselves—and from a Power greater than myself.

—Your User[2]

The second letter, which encourages parents to avoid codependent, enabling traps, is a letter from a parent to her child. This is a letter that a mother wrote when she was well on her way in her journey toward empowerment. She describes how she was before she started treatment:

When my son was using, I was "Queen of the Roller Coaster Ride." My life was quite unmanageable. But I wanted help, and I was ready to ask.

She and her son were treated for a year, and when he graduated from his program, she read this letter to him:

Dear son,

This is a letter of emancipation for you and for me. I am freeing you from being enabled by me to think that the world should grant your every wish. I am being freed to have a relationship with you based on mutual love and respect, not manipulation and power struggles.

I will no longer attempt to solve your problems by running interference for you with treatment staff, teachers, principals, or others. I will also refrain from offering unsolicited advice and solutions.

I will no longer allow you to manipulate me through demands, angry outbursts, or being dragged into explanations and debates.

I will not provide for everything you want, but don't need. I will allow you the opportunity to earn those things for yourself.

I will have faith in your ability to make good choices for yourself.

I will have respect for your ability to accept responsibility for the consequence of your choices.

I will be honest about my feelings.

With love and respect,

Mom

Taking care of yourself

This is a difficult chapter to read and respond to because it deals with the pain, loneliness, and manipulations that are so common in families with drug/alcohol abusers. Therefore, it is especially important that you nurture yourself while you contemplate what is written:

- Look for books, films, and tapes mentioned in Appendix A. For example, you could go to a large bookstore to look for these authors. Wander the aisles and pay attention to the soothing music that often exists in such places. Check out Nature Solitude CDs or tapes in the store. With these recordings, you can be on a nature walk while you are in your car, doing housework, or when you are reading Al-Anon, Nar-Anon, or Families Anonymous material. Go to the travel section and browse through a few books about locations you would like to visit some day. You need to have focused ways to dream and to relax as a way to nurture yourself. Have a cup of coffee or tea with a chocolate-chip cookie or a scone in the coffee bar. Lose yourself in this experience. Have fun with it.

- Exercise helps relieve tension and elevate your mood. It also promotes healthier eating and can even help you sleep better. It is important to build some daily exercise into your life if it isn't there already. You can start small with a ten-minute walk. You don't want to beat yourself up by setting a goal that is so high you can't complete it. Taking care of yourself is easier when your body has a way to get rid of pain and frustration through a walk, working on some machines in a gym, running on the treadmill you have in your bedroom, or swimming some laps. Remember, you're worth it. Exercise will also help you reduce rage attacks, depression, and low self-esteem.

- Check the literature table at your Al-Anon, Nar-Anon, or Families Anonymous meeting. Material is free or at cost. This would be a good time to purchase the daily reading book *One Day at a Time* (Al-Anon) or *Today a Better Way* (Families Anonymous). Notice at the end of each book that there is an index with page numbers related to the topics family members usually struggle with in terms of the consequences of living with a drug/alcohol abuser. When you are having a particular struggle, you can turn to these pages for support. Many parents recommend that you keep material like this to read in the bathroom; you can lock yourself in when your teenager is hounding you and emerge serene.

- Parents who relate to the deep pain described in this chapter find that individual therapy or a treatment program is often a helpful supplement to support group meetings like Nar-Anon, Families Anonymous, or Al-Anon. Therapists with the specialty of helping those struggling with codependency issues can be social workers, psychologists, or chemical dependency treatment professionals in private practice. Ask at your support group meeting for ideas on good therapists.

- Refer to Appendix A's "Adolescent treatment programs" section for a representative list of treatment programs that may help you. You can also check for similar programs in your community.

CHAPTER 7

Communication and Relationships

'Twas brillig, and the slithy toves
Did gyre and gimble in the wabe
All mimsy were the borogoves,
And the mome raths outgrabe.

—Lewis Carroll
Jabberwocky

CODEPENDENCY COMPLICATES our emotional and physical health and our relationships with others. If we do not address our painful feelings directly, a natural consequence is that we communicate with and through our defenses. We can easily push others away with these defenses and complicate our loneliness even further. This chapter will discuss defenses that increase loneliness, the characteristic ways that families of substance abusers communicate, unhealthy roles that family members play to cope with the pain of drug/alcohol abuse, and what to do to get help.

Defenses and communication

The following anonymously-written list of attitudes that increase loneliness has been making the rounds at many Al-Anon meetings. The list typifies the chip-on-the-shoulder attitude that parents often try to change as the first step to making changes in their lives. The list is one of the best examples of the types of defensive attitudes that lead to poor communication with others. As you read it, think about what it would be like for you if you knew people who presented themselves in this way. Keep in mind that the unknown author of these twelve steps is using them to parallel the Twelve Steps of recovery, or health, which we will discuss in more depth in Chapter 8, *Working on Recovery*.

Twelve Steps to a Relapse

1. I decided I could handle my emotional problems if other people would just quit trying to run my life.

2. I firmly believe that there is no greater power than myself, and anyone who says different is insane.

3. I made a decision to remove my will and my life from God who didn't understand me anyhow.

4. I made a searching and thorough moral inventory of everyone I knew so they couldn't fool me and take advantage of my good nature.

5. I sought these people out and tried to get them to admit to me, by God, the exact nature of their wrongs.

6. I became willing to help these people get rid of these defects of character.

7. I was humble enough to ask these people to remove their shortcomings.

8. I kept a list of all the people who had harmed me, and waited patiently for a chance to get even.

9. I got even with these people whenever possible, except when to do so would get me in trouble.

10. I continue to take everyone's inventory and when they are wrong, which is most of the time, I promptly make them admit it.

11. I sought through the concentration of my will power to get God to see that my ideas were best and all I needed was the power to carry them out.

12. Having maintained my emotional strength for many years with these steps, I can thoroughly recommend them to others who wish to be left alone.

Unfortunately, individuals who relate this way to others are often the very same people who complain that no one listens to them. They think they have the answer for everything, so they resent this lack of respect for their solutions. They are often consumed with blaming others for their problems and moods, and they are filled with self-pity. You may find them very difficult to converse with because they want to go on and on about how they qualify for martyrdom.

These are often the communication patterns of parents who bring their teenagers to an assessment and/or treatment. These ways of communicating are often the results of emotional burnout. They are the attitudes of "the rock" in the Simon and Garfunkel song discussed in Chapter 5, *Working on Your Feelings*.

The feelings and behavior chart in Table 6-1 in Chapter 6, *Harmful Consequences from Normal Feelings*, focused on how substance abusers' inside feelings are similar to those of their family members. The chart has been expanded in Table 7-1 to show the types of behaviors that family members often choose to deal with their feelings. The troublesome behaviors that present problems with communication include the same self-righteousness, blaming, aggressiveness, anger, controlling of others, abusiveness, grandiosity, and criticism that we observe in drug/alcohol abusers. The similarities are a reminder of how codependency works. The other similarity is how these behaviors are only defenses. Remember, underneath these outside communication patterns are self-hatred, fear, helplessness, hurt, loneliness, feelings of rejection, and low self-worth.

Table 7-1. Characteristics of Substance-Abusing Families

Abuser's True Feelings	Abuser's Behavior	Family Members' Feelings	Family Members' Behavior
Guilt, self-hatred	Self-righteous, blaming	Guilt, self-hatred	Self-righteous, blaming
Fear	Aggressive, angry	Fear	Aggressive, angry
Helplessness	Controlling (others)	Helplessness	Controlling (others)
Hurt	Abusive	Hurt	Abusive
Loneliness	Rejecting, grandiose	Loneliness	Rejecting, grandiose
Low self-worth	Judging, criticizing	Low self-worth	Judging, criticizing

This table shows the behaviors that family members choose to deal with their inner pain. These behaviors can push others away and cause significant communication problems in the family, as illustrated by the parents of teens speaking below:

> *Why couldn't I get my son to listen to what I was saying? It infuriated me that he wouldn't follow the rules. It was so opposite from how I was taught to respect my parents.*

My self-worth was shot because my son didn't respect me. I turned into a raging maniac with all my judging and criticizing. I look back now, and I hardly recognize the person I became.

· · · · ·

In my parents' generation there was no discussion about what we were supposed to do. [In our present circumstances] I felt helpless. I couldn't stop all the power struggles. I felt guilty, and I got very self-righteous and blaming.

· · · · ·

The uncertainty about what was going on made me feel even more helpless. Was it just normal adolescence or something else? But then I was very blaming of everything. It was as if I knew all the answers. That was really the opposite of what I was feeling.

· · · · ·

The chaos and uncertainty of our situation caused difficulties between my wife and me because we had different ways of dealing with things. She was more the intuitive type and could express her feelings. I was more analytical. We were constantly at odds with each other. I thought she was moving too fast, and it seemed like she was much too dramatic. We had a lot of tension between us because we approached things in a different way. We felt really insecure inside, but we were judging and blaming each other for what was going on.

· · · · ·

We started blaming each other about what was going on. But we never said we were lonely like we really were.

· · · · ·

My husband and I lost the ability to communicate without being snappish. I was very lonely.

· · · · ·

The lonelier I got, the more sarcastic I got to my wife. It was really a bad time. We're lucky we didn't get a divorce. We didn't know we had a drug addict in our house. We found out in treatment that we were acting like families usually do in our situation. That was a big relief.

Words from these parents demonstrate how lonely they were during their burnout. Another Simon and Garfunkel song, "The Sound of Silence," speaks of this loneliness with images of walking alone in restless dreams, listening to voices that have no meaning, and seeing neon lights that mock inside pain.

Many parents can relate to sleepless nights tossing and turning in the darkness, their drug-abusing adolescents out on the streets after a fight in the living room. Then there is the loneliness of going to work the next morning, their adolescents still missing, and not saying anything about that sleepless night of terror. This silence may be out of fear that colleagues and friends will judge them harshly for their inability to control their teenagers. Sometimes, however, it is because of increased loneliness when outsiders suggest easy solutions to complicated pain. These glib solutions offered by others serve to stifle open communication. The following parents tell of keeping silent:

> However true it is that God does love us, or that it is possible to have a "good day," I was not ready to receive these words until I dealt with my pain. Well-meaning people only made me feel worse. I didn't want to open up about what I was feeling because I thought they would judge me for not being strong.

• • • • •

> I felt really guilty when people said things to me that were meant to be helpful. It wasn't as easy to feel better as they said. And the way they smiled made me feel even worse. It was almost as if they didn't recognize how difficult the situation was for me. They were trying to help and that made me feel lonelier. What they were saying made me want to get away from them.

> If only someone had encouraged me to cry. I even felt guilty when I was by myself, and I did cry. I had so much pain bottled up inside. I needed someone who wasn't put off by tears.

Parents are able to feel less lonely when others relate to what they are feeling, or point them to a resource that can validate their sense of despair. The following two parents found some solace when spiritual leaders told them to look in particular places in the Bible, so they didn't feel cut off from "normal" human experience:

When my son began treatment for drug abuse, I had a lot of pain and loneliness. A lot of my pain was related to feeling angry with God that this was happening in my family. I talked to my pastor, and he told me more about the psalms. I hadn't realized that a lot of them are complaints about what is happening. He told me that God understands, that you can be angry with Him. It's okay to question His love when bad things are happening.

I felt so relieved. I was getting tired of all those easy solutions. I needed to work through my pain. Now I have an even deeper faith. It's like God was patient with me. He was there with me all along.

· · · · ·

I was so lonely when our daughter went to addiction treatment. I felt that God left me to deal with it by myself. I was angry. The pastor at our church told me to look again at the passages about Job. My faith in God really deepened after that. Job was an angry man, but God hung in there with him. It was okay for me to struggle.

Common family roles

It is common for family members to feel spiritually adrift and to have anger, loneliness, and despair when there is substance abuse in the family. Family members also tend to adjust to their pain, confusion, and isolation by taking on certain roles to cope with their distress. The mother of a drug-abusing teen describes an experience common to many families:

Everyone in our family was a mess. It was a living hell to be in the same house together. When I look back now, I can only feel sad at how lonely we all were. But we treated each other like we were characters in Lord of the Flies. *It was like we were trying to kill each other on that island.*

Research and clinical experience with families under duress have shown that when there is drug/alcohol abuse within the family, the family members take on characteristic communication styles or patterns of behavior, often referred to as family roles. Roles vary for each family member because of personality differences. The various roles play off each other, complement each other, and maintain equilibrium in a type of organized pattern or system, like the parts of a mobile positioned to balance each other's weight.

Individual roles are explained more fully in the sections that follow, but, briefly, the names of the roles are:

- Drug/alcohol Abuser Teenager
- Super Parent
- Prosecutor
- Family Hero
- Lost Child
- Mascot
- Scapegoat (also called rebellious child)

Not all families have every role represented. For example, if a teen alcoholic is an only child, just the first three roles might be seen. In a family with three children, each sibling of the abuser child might take one of the remaining roles based on a number of factors, such as temperament.

The concept of the family as a system grew out of research on families of schizophrenics in the 1950s, which are described in a fascinating book about healing families, *The Family Crucible*, written by renowned experts in the family therapy field, Augustus Y. Napier, PhD, and Carl A. Whitaker, MD. In their chapter "The Concept of the System," they write:

> Through this research, the scientists began to think of the family in a new way. Rather than look at it as a collection of individuals, they began to view the family as having almost the same kind of organized integrity that the biological organism has. The family functioned as an entity, as a "whole," with its own structure and rules. . . .
>
> These parts [behaved] in a predictable relationship with one another, thus creating a pattern that maintained a stable equilibrium by making changes in itself.[1]

Do family members know they are taking on these roles to balance their dysfunction? No. Are these roles predictable? Yes. One parent relates:

> When we went into treatment for our son, it was amazing to me how similar all the families were. I had thought that we were the only family that acted in the unhealthy ways we did. It was amazing how we had all fallen into certain roles. Our counselor kept telling us that we were normal. That was such a relief. We weren't off the deep end like I thought.

The next two sections explain common roles assumed by members of a family in which there is drug or alcohol abuse. Notice that there are certain visible qualities with each role and certain inner feelings. Also, each role represents something different to each member of the family. Each role, with treatment, has a hopeful future; without help, each has an unhappy future.

Substance abuser and parental roles

The first role to examine is that of the Drug/alcohol Abuser Teenager. As we discussed earlier, this adolescent often appears self-righteous, aggressive, angry, rigid, and highly critical of others. They are filled with shame, guilt, fear, pain and self-doubt. To the family, they represent "the problem," most likely because of their constant mood changes. Without help, the abuser's future may be death; with help, they can reach their potential. These drug/alcohol abuser teens, now sober in recovery, describe their mood swings, how they treated their families abusively, and how they really felt underneath. They illustrate the problem in communication when defenses are used instead of true feelings:

> I blamed my mom for all the troubles I was having because she was so hard on me about my grades and my friends. But I knew that I was failing in school and in the beginning I had a lot of shame about that. I never talked about it, though. I wanted to use drugs, and my mom was on my case, so it was easier to blame her for everything than talk about my feelings.

· · · · ·

> I used a lot of anger on my brother to make sure that he didn't tell what was going on. I threatened that I would hurt him, and he was afraid of me. I also said that if he told that meant he didn't love me. I told him in treatment that I was sorry I treated him like that. Now that I am in recovery, I feel embarrassed about it. I want my brother to look up to me in positive ways.

The anger and intimidation used by these teens presents challenges to the rest of their families. To keep balance, one or the other parent usually plays the next two roles whether they are married or not. In single-parent households, there is often a grandparent who plays one of the roles.

The Super Parent or Super Grandparent is often the most understanding and gullible person in terms of how they are seen by drug/alcohol abuser adolescents. They are often the chief enablers. They appear as though they can handle everything, and they often present themselves as cheerful. Underneath, however, they often feel guilty that there is nothing they can do to prevent what is happening. They feel inadequate, hurt, and angry. It is easy for them to blame every person, place, or thing that they believe to be the cause of the problems in the home, but they tend to excuse the out-of-control teenager. Examples of enabling and codependency given in Chapter 6 illustrate the lengths to which sweet Super Parents or Super Grandparents will go in a perceived positive direction for the family.

Unfortunately, this enabling creates hostility in those in the contrasting role, which is often called the Prosecutor. Those who take the prosecutor role also feel inadequate, confused, and guilty, but they express these feelings by lecturing, criticizing, and preaching—which often leads to threatening, intimidating, and, sometimes, abusive behavior. They are usually the ones who are the most suspicious of drug/alcohol abusers. They are also the least enabling. Sadly, the prosecutor focuses the family anger. Everyone is angry with the out-of-control household they live in, but prosecutors are so angry they become more the focus than the drug/alcohol abusers themselves.

The following parents and grandparents relate how their contrasting roles played off each other and increased their loneliness and isolation. Their experiences are common:

My wife and I played these contrasting roles. The more one of us did our thing, the more extreme was the other's reaction.

. . . . .

I was really furious that my husband believed all the lies my son told him. I told him how incompetent he was as a father. He only clammed up more after that, and that made me even more furious. I was really afraid of what was going on, but instead of saying that, I acted like a real bitch and only pushed him away further. Our family counselor helped us to see that we were both trying to stop an out-of-control situation, so we needed to forgive each other and move on. I have also had to work on forgiving myself for how I acted.

. . . . .

My mother was the epitome of the sweet grandmother. The easier she was on the kids, the more I felt I had to come down hard. That was really difficult because I was fighting against my own mother.

Others describe further how conflict impacted their relationships:

My grandson had a sad life. After all, his father left when he was five. I couldn't understand why my daughter was so hard on him. All those rules! I didn't need rules at my house. We got along great. Then I realized he was stealing money from me and having parties when I was away. I had a difficult time saying no to him. He took advantage of that. It was hard between my daughter and me because we had been so different with him. I had to learn to have rules, too. My daughter and I had counseling together to get our relationship back on track.

• • • • •

I called my wife the "Gestapo Queen." I got more and more sarcastic about her rules or her concerns about my son and that would make things even worse. Of course, the kids loved the fact that I was with them against her. I didn't even think about how lonely she was. It never occurred to me by the way she was acting. We had a lot of work to do on our relationship when our son went into treatment. I definitely had to work on my sarcasm.

• • • • •

It's like our relationship was in a taffy pull. My wife and I were at two extremes pulling, and our relationship fell on the floor.

• • • • •

I understand now how lonely my wife and I were. But we never said it at the time. There was so much uncertainty about what was going on, and we each handled it in different ways. We were both very isolated.

The sibling response

While parents are polarized in the ways they communicate, brothers and sisters of drug/alcohol abusing teenagers also cope by taking on certain roles. The first of these is the Family Hero.

Children who take on the behaviors of the Family Hero try to balance out the dysfunction caused by substance abusers by reinforcing the families' feelings of self-worth. Those who fall easily into this role are high achievers. They earn good grades with persistent effort, are often involved in school activities, and appear to have many friends. They receive praise within the family and from aunts, uncles, and grandparents. They appear as the hero in the family, in direct contrast to the problem child.

Beneath this facade, however, family heroes often feel inadequate. To help the family, they are also trying to change the behavior of the drug/alcohol abuser. Tension between them is high; chemical abusers resent all the positive attention heroes are receiving, and they also resent how the heroes try to change them. Therefore, attempts at rehabilitation are met with defiance and sarcasm. A teen who took on the role of Family Hero discusses the common feelings of isolation:

> *My sister was so out of control with her friends and her using, and I really felt sorry for my parents. What was happening was especially hard on my mom. I hated to see her cry so much. At least she was happy that I had good grades and wasn't getting into trouble. I felt proud when I heard someone praise her for being a good mother.*
>
> *I felt really lonely inside because the better I did the more my sister called me a geek and made fun of me. I couldn't tell my mom about this because she had enough to worry about. And I sure didn't want to talk about it with my friends. I wanted them to like my sister. I thought that maybe she would turn around if she hung out with my friends and me.*

These words show typical pressures that are felt by those in the role of Family Hero. Not only are they trying to provide relief to those with the most pain in the family, they are also desperate to rehabilitate the abuser/alcoholic/ addict. It is easy to see that they lose focus on themselves and their own needs. Their self-esteem is often based on others in the family doing well, and they feel responsible when this does not happen. They communicate their inside loneliness and pain by working harder for change. This is futile, however, because they cannot change others, particularly the substance abuser. They can also start acting like the prosecutor and being bossy and arrogant in the way they try to implement change. This alienates them from everyone else in the family.

It is easy to see that the family heroes, without treatment, can grow up to be workaholics who feel responsible for every organization they work for and every person who works within it. Just as they took over responsibilities for the substance abusers in their families, they can be manipulated into staying late to finish other people's work. They can also feel guilty when they are tired or when they go home with projects left unfinished on their desk, even when these projects do not have to be completed for weeks. On the other hand, when the inside pain and loneliness of family heroes is addressed, they can learn to accept failure and that they are not responsible for the positive outcome of every situation. They also have the organizational and leadership qualities that make for good executives.

In contrast to the visibly successful Family Hero is the invisible Lost Child. These quiet children are the ones who seem to withdraw into their own world. They often feel rejected and inadequate. They are often the children who have hung back from conflict and been more passive and easy in temperament since they were in the crib. When there is major conflict in their families with something like drug/alcohol abuse, they tend to fade further and further into the background. It is as if they lose their personality. As a children's art therapist explains:

> The passive or lost child in a family will often draw themselves without a head or a leg or with one of these hidden behind a tree. Their pencil lines are also very light and tentative. The lost child feels like they are not a whole person in the family, and they are powerless to make a difference. Their loneliness and isolation are intense.

These children are followers who have a great deal of difficulty making decisions. They can be a relief to their families because they represent one less child to worry about. They are very fragile, however, and are at high risk for pregnancy or being on the receiving end of an abusive relationship. They do not have the skills to assert themselves in order to leave an unhealthy situation. Also, they are so needy of attention and love that they cannot discriminate between a good relationship and an unhealthy one.

These children are often very creative and find relief in drawing or storytelling to their dolls or other toys. With help from a therapist to talk about their feelings during this painful period in their lives, they can maximize their potential. Without help, they are at high risk to have continued problems such as being unable to care for their own children, choosing weak partners, and being unable to separate from these unhealthy, abusive relationships.

The Mascots also have behaviors that represent relief for their families. These are the children who are the charmers, the ones whose comic behavior relieves family tension. They are also the children who are unable to deal with their pain honestly and, however funny they can be, their behaviors keep others at a distance. Some of the most gifted comedians have developed their skills by adjusting to a painful childhood through entertaining others. On the other hand, their humor often shows anger and sarcasm, and the feelings of loneliness and isolation may only intensify if they are unable to communicate their pain more directly. An experienced family therapist describes how humor can be a mechanism hiding darker emotions:

> The comic child is often deep in denial about what is going on unless you can get them to stop cracking jokes. This is difficult to do, however, because they like to be center-stage, and they ward off attempts to be serious. These are often the kids that get sent to the principal because they disrupt the class. But they will not easily admit to being lonely or scared at home. It's as if their whole world will fall apart if they get serious.

If these children do not get help with communicating their painful feelings, they can remain immature and have continued difficulty handling stress. They are at high risk for becoming drug/alcohol abusers as a way to loosen up even further to escape their pain. With help, they can discard their compulsive need for attention and be more open about their pain and disappointment when life events merit such responses. Their capacity for true intimacy will also increase when they lessen the distance that humor often provides.

The last role that is often identified in families where there is pain associated with drug/alcohol abuse or dependency is that of the Scapegoat or Rebellious Child. These children communicate their pain by rebelling, challenging rules, and fighting. Sometimes they take the spotlight away from the drug/alcohol abusers and mask the abuser's problems even further. They may also be abusing chemicals. Younger children who have this role are very difficult to reach because the attention in school or at home is so often on their disruptive behaviors, and they may not talk about their painful feelings. A children's art therapist describes how art therapy can help these children open up:

> Art therapy can be a very helpful tool for the aggressive, rebellious child because they put energy in their art with angry, bold lines. Then we can talk about the monsters they have created in their pictures. It is safer for them to talk about how a monster scares them than to talk directly about someone in their family. Their rebellion is a way to gain mastery over their fears. When they can talk this through with a therapist, they can lessen the rebellion and talk more openly about what is going on.

Parents from dysfunctional families

What if parents are adult children of alcoholics or grew up in dysfunctional homes? How will this affect the roles they take on and the ways they communicate when their children are displaying the behaviors of drug/alcohol abusers?

If parents grew up in homes where there was alcohol abuse or other high-stress problems, it will be normal for them to revert to childhood roles during the high stress of their children's chemical abuse. For example, it is common for parents who were the family hero as children to try to control and organize the present situation. The mother of an addict explains how she tried to retain control over her family situation:

> I was the responsible oldest child growing up in an alcoholic and abusive family and was very good at organizing us four kids to get out of danger. I even orchestrated a runaway across town when I was seven. My brothers and sister thought of me as the mother all the time we were living at home.
>
> When my 17-year-old son started getting into trouble, I was right on him. He covered up his drug use so we didn't know that was the problem, but I sensed that he was lying a lot of the time. I didn't trust him, and it drove me nuts how gullible my husband was to all the manipulations. I was really overwhelmed by what was happening, and very lonely. I went into high gear, however, so it looked like I was confident. My anxiety about our out-of-control situation was motivating me to take charge and get us out of danger.
>
> I never told anyone how lonely I felt, and I only used defenses, so no one could get close to me. I alienated everyone in my family by telling them all what to do, so I really deserved the title of Gestapo Queen. I was obnoxious, no doubt about it.
>
> As I look back, I felt responsible because things were not changing. It was like I had failed the family because I couldn't make things right. Actually, it was a relief when we found out that our son was an addict. I cried going down in the elevator when we checked him into treatment because I was so glad that someone else could take over and help us. I was a wreck from trying so hard and getting nowhere.

Behaving in high gear as the family hero helped this mother feel competent and, most of all, lessened her fear and anxiety. But the price that she paid was very high. Also, she was unable to communicate her inside feelings. She trapped herself in her pain.

Two parents who played another role growing up also illustrate how parents can revert to old roles when their child is abusing drugs:

> *I hung in the background when I was a boy and didn't say much when my father was abusive and acting like a practicing alcoholic. I also copied my mother who kept the peace by giving in. When my son was so out of control, I did the same thing. But I never talked about how lonely and scared I felt as a child, and in our current situation, until we went to family treatment.*

· · · · ·

> *Things were so out of control when I was a girl, but it was my sister who spoke up, not me. I just watched and withdrew into myself. I was overwhelmed and lonely, but I created a fantasy life that had a lot of denial in it. When my son started getting into trouble, I felt the same overwhelmed and lonely feelings. And I created a fantasy life all over again. I saw him the way I wanted to see him. I made excuses for everything he did. I was the lost child all over again.*

These roles, and others, usually represent an extension of an adult's healthy personality. Under stress, however, the roles can become unhealthy and highly dysfunctional. The family heroes, for example, can become over-organized, over-controlling, and highly judgmental if family members don't respond to their leadership. They often feel that their inability to make things right means that they are bad persons. To counteract this painful feeling, they often become more rigid to control the chaos. The lost children, for their response, usually feel helpless to do anything and become increasingly passive and withdrawn.

This conflict of roles affects the strength of parenting teams. Withdrawal of the lost child parent aggravates the controlling behavior of the family hero parent and vice versa. Children are not only afraid that their parents are falling apart; they are afraid of the often vicious arguing that goes on between these two adults. The children then revert to, and strengthen, their own roles as a way of coping with their pain. But *no one* is talking about his true feelings of fear, anxiety, helplessness, and isolation. Communication has deteriorated into false roles that say "stay away from me." Everyone's defenses are increasingly rigid and impenetrable so that others do stay away. The isolation only gets worse.

Solutions—what can be done?

The family situations described earlier seemed hopeless. No one was communicating her true feelings. Everyone felt lonely and afraid.

Things cannot get better unless there is change. But what can be done?

As a first step to improve lack of communication and restore family health, family members need to understand what is going on. Predictably, parents feel crazy, out of control, and even suicidal as the family disease progresses. By understanding this process, the ongoing role-playing, and the fear and loneliness experienced by all family members, parents can start to feel normal. This restored sense of being normal can provide the hope and energy to get help. A father comments:

> When my wife and I brought our son to treatment, I had so much shame because I thought that we had caused his drug dependency. After all, the way we were living was horrible. I was sure that this had driven my son to addiction. We learned right away that the communication problems were a result of his drug dependency, not the cause. We also learned how normal we were, and how other families were just like us. I felt really energized to start working on undoing the damage that had been done, to start communicating with my true feelings. When we understood what had been going on, it was like opening a window. The fresh air felt great for all of us. We could start over.

In order to respond effectively to the hopelessness and despair of the family under stress, professionals need to understand the family disease process. Parents in treatment often wish that outside professionals had raised the possibility of drug/alcohol abuse during earlier stages in a progression. Instead, professionals often overlook this possibility.

Looking back, parents also can feel angry at school professionals who did not recognize the signs and symptoms of alcohol/drug abuse and dependency and who were fooled by kids complaining about poor communication at home. Many school districts do fine work in early identification of alcohol/drug problems and have trained staff well in how not to be manipulated by teenagers, but this manipulation can still happen. A guidance counselor who learned her lesson relates how one student misled her:

> I got totally pulled in by a kid. I knew he had problems with alcohol, but he told me stories about his parents that made them look horrible. I thought that I would drink, too, if I had parents like that. I am embarrassed to say that I think I said this to the kid, and that was really bad. He had an assessment, however, and he was middle-stage alcohol dependency.

> He had really used me. I was too gullible and didn't know enough about the signs and symptoms of the disease.

On the other hand, as an assessment professional explains, having good communication at home can also be a problem in terms of assumptions:

> School professionals can also minimize symptoms of chemical dependency if they think that the teenager comes from a good home. I have had it happen so many times that guidance counselors didn't refer earlier because they thought this. They felt that it would be an insult to the parents to ask if there was a communication problem or if the kid was acting out at home.

> I have to keep educating folk that whether or not kids come from a good home has nothing to do with whether or not they can be addicts or alcoholics. The prejudice about good parents definitely gets in the way of looking at the truth of what is going on.

Taking care of yourself

Given the confusion that can exist in the professional community, it is even more important that parents understand what happens with communication in families when drug/alcohol abuse or dependency is present. The family system is not hopeless and beyond repair. Parents can start to get well by talking with each other about their *inside* feelings.

Parents also need to educate themselves so they can separate from outsiders' judgments and not isolate themselves further from the realities of their lives. This separation may also need to occur with extended family members who do not understand what is going on and are quick to judge.

Many parents relate how easy it is to feel resentful of the professionals and extended family members who misdiagnosed or didn't understand. But, as this mother of a recovering son explains, resentments only hurt you and not the person you resent:

> I heard at an Al-Anon meeting that when I resented someone, I was letting him or her live in my head rent-free. I thought about them all the time, and I even woke up in the middle of the night thinking about them. I made myself miserable while they were off having a good day. When I realized this, I decided that I didn't want to give them all this power to ruin my life in the here and now. I needed to work on how I held on to resentments. They were only hurting me.

Parents who are working on issues discussed in this chapter can:

- Continue to attend meetings where you share with others, such as Al-Anon, Nar-Anon, or Families Anonymous, group therapy for adult children of alcoholics, and meetings held in other support settings.

- Look in Appendix A, *Resources*, for reading that would be helpful. *Loving Each Other: The Challenge of Human Relationships*, by Leo Buscaglia, is a good book on topics in this chapter.

CHAPTER 8

Working on Recovery

All things are difficult before they are easy.

—John Morley

PARENTS WHO BRING their adolescents to an assessment for drug/alcohol abuse and then to addiction treatment will hear the word *recovery* to describe what their teenagers will have to substitute for their using lifestyle. Parents will also be told that they, too, will need to start a program of recovery, and that this program will be similar to what their teenagers are working on.

All of this can be bewildering to parents. How could they be working on the same things as their teenagers? Their teenagers are the ones who need help for their addiction, not them.

This chapter will discuss what is meant by having a program of recovery, where the term came from, the Twelve Steps that are central to any recovery, how early recovery for adolescents and parents differs from later recovery, unique recovery issues when parents are also in AA or NA, and how parents can instill recovery values in their homes. The promises of recovery in the *Big Book of Alcoholics Anonymous* and the Serenity Prayer provide hope and inspiration for recovery, and they will be discussed in "Taking care of yourself," a section at the end of this chapter.

Origins and principles of recovery

Recovery is a word that is used to describe the attitudes and behaviors that are going to be needed to stay clean—that is, off drugs and sober. It is also used to describe what family members work on to heal themselves from the destructive impact of addiction. It is a word that has been written about in many languages since a stockbroker, Bill W., and a physician, Dr. Bob, founded Alcoholics Anonymous in Akron, Ohio, in 1935.

Alcoholics Anonymous and recovery

Bill W. and Dr. Bob founded AA after their repeated attempts to stop drinking on their own. The first AA meeting consisted of these two people, but word spread quickly about the power of self-help support, and the numbers multiplied. The principles of recovery were organized into Twelve Steps and Twelve Traditions, and members of the Akron groups took this recovery message to the nearby city of Cleveland. Word about a new way to stay sober spread quickly to those suffering alcoholics who were desperate for tools to help them become sober. By 1948, 13 years later, 87 individuals and groups had applied for listing in the Directory of Alcoholics Anonymous from locations as diverse as Long Beach, California; Chicago, Illinois; Toronto, Canada; and Richmond, Virginia.[1]

Now AA exists in more than 130 countries. The Twelve Traditions cover group organization, function, anonymity, and relationships within and without the groups and are similar all over the world. At least 225 support groups, including Narcotics Anonymous, Cocaine Anonymous, Emotions Anonymous, Debtors Anonymous, Early-onset Alzheimer's Anonymous, Overeaters Anonymous, Parents Anonymous, Schizophrenics Anonymous, Families Anonymous, and Al-Anon have adopted the principles of the Twelve Step recovery. Some of the early AA meeting places, such as a woman named Hazel's cramped living room in her farmhouse located outside of Minneapolis, have grown into well-known treatment centers (the farmhouse became Hazelden) where these Twelve Steps are at the center of treatment for addicts and their families.

Spreading the word

Stanley E. Gitlow, MD, in his foreword to *The Recovery Book*, describes the early years of Alcoholics Anonymous:

> ...*It became apparent that written explanations of the recovery process were needed for explanation, understanding, and ongoing consistency of the program.*[2]

The *Big Book of Alcoholics Anonymous*, officially titled *Alcoholics Anonymous*, written by the first members of AA, was the first elaborate description of Twelve Step recovery attitudes and behaviors. *The Primer on Alcoholism* followed, written by the first woman in AA, Marty Mann. The same materials from those early years are still used, and widely translated, today.

Since 1935, alcoholics have been acquiring experience, strength, and hope from attending Twelve Step meetings and using the literature that is found at these meetings. The Twelve Steps are read at the beginning, and the rest of the meeting revolves around their interpretation. The Steps have also been adopted by other self-help recovery programs and are used for study and assignments in treatment programs.

The adolescents' recovery will depend on whether or not they accept, and live by, these Steps:

The Twelve Steps[3]

1. *We admitted we were powerless over alcohol—that our lives had become unmanageable.*

2. *Came to believe that a Power greater than ourselves could restore us to sanity.*

3. *Made a decision to turn our will and our lives over to the care of God, as we understood Him.*

4. *Made a searching and fearless moral inventory of ourselves.*

5. *Admitted to God, to ourselves, and to another human being the exact nature of our wrongs.*

6. *Were entirely ready to have God remove all these defects of character.*

7. *Humbly asked Him to remove our shortcomings.*

8. *Made a list of all persons we had harmed, and became willing to make amends to them all.*

9. *Made direct amends to such people wherever possible except when to do so would injure them or others.*

10. *Continued to take personal inventory and when we were wrong, promptly admitted it.*

11. *Sought through prayer and meditation to improve our conscious contact with God, as we understood Him, praying only for knowledge of His will for us and the power to carry that out.*

12. *Having had a spiritual awakening as a result of these Steps, we tried to carry this message to others and to practice these principles in all our affairs.*

Adolescents and early recovery

When adolescent addicts/alcoholics enter treatment for the first time, their level of denial about their disease is usually very high. This complicates their recovery. The first three Steps help them with the foundation they will need to remain sober and drug-free.

Step One

The First Step asks adolescents to admit to themselves that their drug/alcohol-using lives are unmanageable because using has led to repeated harmful consequences. In addition, this Step asks them to admit to themselves that they are alcoholics and addicts who cannot control their use by will power alone; they need to surrender to the principles of a program of recovery. They need to give up their powerful egos.

This is a difficult Step for all addicts/alcoholics. Denial, delusion, and rationalization fuel addiction. Addicts/alcoholics must free themselves of these if they are to take their First Step and begin recovery. Adolescent addicts share stories about how difficult this process can be. Each story illustrates problems with denial, delusion, and rationalization:

> The hardest part for me at the beginning was admitting to myself the insanity of things I had done as a result of my drug-using lifestyle.

> When I was told in my first treatment that I needed to quit using because of my consequences, I thought that the problem was that I got caught. I focused more on that than what the consequences were in the first place. I thought the whole thing about my life being unmanageable was a joke. I wasn't that bad. I decided to go along with what I had to do to get by, and get out of treatment, but I had no intention of quitting.

· · · · ·

> I went to my first rehab to save myself from going to jail, but I had no intention of working a program of recovery when I got out. I told myself that my drug of choice was the problem. I could just use something else, and I would be okay. I would just use to socialize and that's all. When I left treatment, I was told not to hang around my old friends, but I did anyway. They had drugs waiting for me. I convinced myself that using my drug of choice again would be okay.

I really didn't take what the counselors said seriously even though I cooperated in my first treatment and did all the assignments. It wasn't a very good program, and they thought I was the star client. They said that my future was jail or death. I didn't believe them. When I went back to jail again for possession and prostitution, I wished that I had listened.

Adolescent addicts/alcoholics need to admit that their life is unmanageable if they are going to turn around their destructive lives. This involves surrendering to an inability to control the use of drugs and alcohol. Two recovering addicts/alcoholics describe the common struggle with surrender:

When I got out of residential treatment after a month and went into outpatient, I thought that I could control my use and hang around my using friends even though I had signed a contract saying certain friends were off limits. I would just lie, but it wouldn't matter because I wouldn't have any problems anyway.

Then I got into a situation where drugs were available. I thought I could just try using and stop, but it didn't work that way. I was right back to where I was before I went to residential treatment. I even got back to the lying, being abusive in my family, getting out of control.

What I see is when I let my big ego get in the way about what I can control, I get right back to using. I have to constantly remind myself of my First Step. Drugs are more powerful than I am. I can't use, and if I do, my life gets unmanageable. Sounds simple, but it is really hard for an addict.

• • • • •

When I got out of treatment the first time, I knew I had a problem with crack cocaine, and I needed to work a recovery program around that. They told me in treatment that I couldn't use other mood-altering chemicals either, but I didn't believe them. How could drinking be a problem? I didn't even enjoy it. I would never be an alcoholic. Drinking had nothing to do with using cocaine.

I started drinking around my friends, then I started drinking by myself. In a single afternoon or evening, I would watch TV by myself and drink a 12- or even a 24-pack. Pretty soon I was right back to using crack cocaine. But this time I didn't snort it; I smoked it. I told myself that smoking it wouldn't be as bad; I wouldn't have the consequences like I did before.

That progressed, and I was right back to snorting it again. I started stealing money from everyone in my family, from stores, from other people on the street. It wasn't just money, but anything I could trade off for crack. Then I realized that if I got caught stealing, I would just waste time in jail and not be able to use, so I started to do what was easier, prostitution.

I had no problem on the streets. Men would pull over day and night. After I asked them if they were cops, and to show me why not, I would get paid for what they wanted and do it. Easy money. I would even steal more from them sometimes. I needed about $400 a day to support my habit.

I started hating myself for what I was doing, and some of the men even tried to get me help. I finally did get busted. I am lucky that I'm not dead, or that I don't have AIDS.

I feel sad when I give this story because it's so pathetic. I'm in treatment again, this time in a good program that knows my manipulations. I see how much I lied to myself about what I was doing. I wasn't willing to admit that I was powerless over drugs and alcohol. I was in so much denial. I wasn't willing to humble myself and admit that drugs were more powerful than I was. I made all these promises about what I wouldn't do, and I couldn't keep any of them. My life was even worse after relapsing, and I'm sorry I didn't pay attention the first time I had a chance.

Now I am working hard to develop a strong recovery program. People say I'm worth recovery and I believe it. I want to be a drug counselor someday so I can help other people like me.

Addicts and alcoholics can struggle with the First Step throughout their lives. Relapse may occur when addicts/alcoholics resume the denial, delusion, and rationalization about their drug/alcohol use and consequences from that use. Parents struggle with this fact because they know, realistically, that relapse can lead to death. It is not something to take lightly. On the other hand, it is also something parents cannot control. An experienced adolescent treatment counselor describes her experiences with relapse and what she advises parents:

During my 30 years of working with teenage addicts, I have seen a lot of relapse. For some kids, it is a rather superficial relapse where they don't take much, and they have such a bad experience with it that they have an even stronger commitment to their recovery afterwards.

On the other hand, I have gone to four funerals of kids who had entered recovery and [then] used only once or twice, but what they used killed them. I also know a young woman who entered recovery, but she relapsed on LSD and her brain got so scrambled that she will never be the same again.

Knowing about the possibility of relapse can be devastating for parents. The binge drinking and the drugs out there today are cause for anyone to be alarmed. On the other hand, our young people are the only ones who can control the choices they make to relapse. We can pray that they don't, of course, but we need to get strong in our own recoveries. If they do decide to relapse, we need to be strong enough to deal with this.

Steps Two and Three

When adolescent addicts/alcoholics realize that their big egos have led them back to using, they are ready to admit that without the help of a power outside themselves, they will not remain sober. They cannot do it by themselves. They will need help if recovery is going to happen.

It is difficult for omnipotent adolescents to admit they need help. An addict who is early in recovery explains how Step Two work begins:

I knew that I had to ask others for help in order to get well, and that was really hard for me. In early treatment, I was told to start small and to just ask my fellow addicts in-group to help. In order to do that, however, I had to be honest about myself. I had this big con going that I wasn't like the others—I was better than them. They couldn't help me. I had to really humble myself, let go of my big ego.

The next assignment was to ask my family for help and to recognize that they had something to offer. This was hard because I had justified my use by telling myself that I had bad parents. This wasn't true, but I wanted to believe it because then I didn't have to take responsibility for my behavior. I could blame it all on them. It made it harder to blame them if they had something good to offer me. I didn't want to humble myself with them.

Recovering addicts/alcoholics in their early 30s who started their recovery when they were teenagers relate their struggles with Step One and Step Two and how giving up their egos helped them:

When I was 17 and in early recovery, I had a hard time with the assignment that I was supposed to get a sponsor in AA to help me. I was told that the best sponsors are those who have a lot of recovery. They are tough, and you know you will learn something from them.

I wanted a young person who was cool, and I think I hoped that this person would be easy on me if I relapsed. I wasn't sure if I wanted to quit or not, and I certainly didn't want some old timer who had all those years telling me what to do. I had a huge ego. I didn't want to listen to anyone but myself.

I dragged my feet for so long that I never asked anyone. One day my counselor said that I had to stand up during announcements at that night's AA meeting and say that I needed a temporary sponsor if anyone would be willing. Someone came up to me when the meeting was over and volunteered. He had been in recovery for over 25 years, and he said that he wanted to help me. I wasn't too happy about it, but he was tough on me and I really needed that, especially in the early days. The way I was going with my big ego, I never would have stayed sober by myself. I am grateful now, especially because I have been sober for almost 15 years.

· · · · ·

When I was first in treatment at 16, I thought I was going to stay straight, but when I got out I didn't listen to my sponsor or do any of the readings or hang out with any new friends. I believed that I could control my use. I started hanging around my old friends, and I was basically saying that I was going to do it my way. I was right back to being my own higher power. I relapsed after three months of this. I was right back to using more than I had planned, being miserable.

I went into treatment a second time and really had to humble myself. I saw where my big ego had gotten me, however, and I worked hard on Step Two and Step Three. If I was going to have recovery, I had to let go of my will. I saw how miserable I was by trying to do it my own way, and that was sort of like a spiritual awakening for me. I couldn't be in control.

I kept having these experiences of when I would try things my way that didn't work. I kept seeing through my consequences that my thinking and my choices were getting me nowhere.

The Twelve Steps were like a power greater than myself that were telling me what to do that was different from my old ways of self-gratification, selfishness, the call of drugs and alcohol, and doing the immoral and unethical things I did in order to get drugs and alcohol.

In recovery, the Steps are there as a guide to give you another perspective. Then you have the AA or NA meetings, the fellowship, the readings you find on the literature table at meetings, your sponsor. All of it is a power greater than yourself that is helping you have recovery and keeping you away from the insanity of your using. I also used prayer and helped other people who were struggling to stay straight, which was kind of like a spiritual experience for me in that I got more back than I gave.

I have been sober for almost 18 years now, but I still remember what those struggles with my ego were like when I was 16. I think there is a lot of hope for addicts if they surrender their egos and listen to others. As the early founders of AA wrote in the Big Book, *"Rarely have we seen a person fail who has followed our path." So true. Recovery works if you work it.*

Parents and early recovery

The first three Steps are also difficult for parents to accept and to practice. They struggle with the same denial, delusion, and rationalization that undermine recovery in their teenagers.

Step One

Parents need to admit in Step One that they are powerless over the addict/alcoholic and the power of alcohol and other mood-altering chemicals in their children's lives. They also have to surrender to the fact that their lives have been unmanageable. Parents of adolescent addicts/alcoholics relate to how difficult it can be to admit powerlessness and unmanageability. Each story describes a common struggle:

When my son and I first came to treatment, I was asked to focus on the First Step. I took home a study sheet I received in our parent education group, and it asked me to list the various ways my life had become unmanageable during my son's using days. There were things on there like losing sleep, losing weight, losing my temper, not being able to do my job, and missing work because I was sick. That was really hard for me because I thought I had failed anyway. All that assignment seemed to say to me was that I was even more of a loser.

What I realized, however, is that those were the behaviors of someone who would lose their life if they kept going. I was really sick of acting these ways, and I was not going to let my life continue with such drastic consequences from what my son was doing.

I also realized that even though I had been a wreck, it didn't matter because my son kept using anyway. His disease was more powerful than I was. I had been unmanageable for nothing. No good came out of it, and I was a wreck besides.

I felt free when I finally accepted the First Step. My parent group counselor was right when she said that the First Step assignment would help me, but I sure didn't want to do it at the beginning.

· · · · ·

The most difficult part of my early recovery was the First Step. It talked about admitting that I was powerless over alcohol, which meant powerless over my son's use of alcohol. Since I spent so much time in trying to get power over what he did, it was difficult to let go of that. It meant to me that I was giving up. That I didn't care. That I didn't love him anymore.

As I worked on the Step, however, I listened for ideas at Al-Anon. I heard how other people worked on it that were farther along than I was. I realized that I was not making any progress by holding this power. I might as well let myself feel powerless and see what happened then.

I began to see that if I spent less time thinking about my son and his future, he had to take responsibility for those things. I learned that he assumed that I would organize his life; I would supply the motivation. I was making him dependent on me for how his life turned out.

He was 17. He wasn't a baby lying in the crib any more. I realized that I was crippling him for the rest of his life. He had to be responsible for his own choices in order to be mature.

It is often difficult for parents to look at the choices they have made in the desire to help their teenagers. They realize that the lectures and angry ultimatums have not worked. These parents describe how they finally surrendered and took their First Step:

> When I started working Step One, I had more time to think about me, and it made me less codependent. I was forced to look at my own choices and at the controlling that was only making my son rebel more. I had been in so many power struggles with him, and when I had to focus on not being able to control him—admitting my powerlessness—he couldn't manipulate me by making my anger one of the excuses he used to run away from his own problems.

· · · · ·

> I finally accepted Step One when I realized that my intelligence and my desire and my strong will could not make my daughter stop using. Also, I had so mismanaged my own life in trying to get her to quit that I lost my job, alienated a lot of my friends, and ended up in a hospital program for stress disorders. I had my own version of insanity, just like my daughter had hers.

· · · · ·

> I thought I had accepted that I was powerless over my son's use of alcohol and drugs, but I still preoccupied myself with what he was doing. I bought into what he would say about how he could control his use, however, and that I shouldn't worry, things would get better. As I look back, I minimized the power of his disease, just like he did. I thought that treatment was just a blip in our lives, and we would go on like we always had. It was almost that my son would be cured; he would get over all this.

> Then he started relapsing and things were going downhill again. Whatever energy I put into his drug problem wasn't helping. This was hard for me because I am a take-charge executive, and I am used to implementing changes when I apply my problem-solving skills. I also love my son deeply, and I was desperate to help him turn his life around.

> My turning point was when I went to a funeral home for a wake to support the family of a colleague's son who had died of a drug overdose. He was in his early 30s, and the family described him as bright, loving, and a wonderful father to his little son. I looked at him in the open casket, and, for the first time, I really felt the power of addiction. He had a lot of the same strengths that my son has. He lost his life because of the

power of his addiction. I started to realize on an emotional level what my own son was up against.

The next day we had family group at our treatment center. We were just sitting there with all the other families when my wife prompted me to tell my son about the viewing. I didn't want to talk about it, so I glared at her, but something kept me going. I started to speak, but the words would not come. My throat tightened. The room took on an almost surreal feeling. It was a moment frozen in time. I just looked at my son, and I started to cry. I couldn't stop. I don't remember what anyone else was doing even though I have heard that the whole group was crying, too.

That was when I realized on the emotional level that I was powerless over alcohol and drugs. I had so much pain.

None of my family, including my wife of twenty years, had ever seen me cry. My son was startled that his use could mean that much to me. I have heard that he has talked a lot about it in his own treatment.

Before that, my intellectualizing with him didn't really mean anything. It was just another lecture. Now he is taking more responsibility for the consequences of his use on others. The important thing for me, though, is that I finally understand this disease and that I can't cure my son. It is clear to him, and to me, that he is responsible for his choices. I also understand what he is up against in trying to work his recovery. I can respect him more. I think he appreciates this.

Steps Two and Three

Like their children in recovery, parents learn that they need more than their own will and intelligence to restore sanity to their lives—that is, to successfully complete a program of recovery. They also need a power outside of themselves, greater than themselves. Part of the difficulty in accepting these Steps is related to confusion over what is meant by power greater than themselves. Parents of adolescent alcoholics/addicts comment on how they resolved this confusion:

As time moved along in my early recovery, I realized that I was not only going to have to give up power over my alcoholic [child], but also over thinking that I alone could solve my own problems. I was confused about what the words "power greater than ourselves" meant, but I knew that I was having problems with my own self-will not working.

I had always been independent, self-reliant. I took great pride in being my own person, a take-charge type. I had to realize that using only my own power, my own will, had gotten me into trouble. I had alienated my son and my wife during my son's use, and my younger children were afraid of my anger. I needed help, but it was hard to ask for it.

· · · · ·

I had always been successful solving problems with my intellect, so it was hard for me to think of coming to believe that a power greater than myself was going to restore me to sanity or that I would turn my will over to a greater power. I had to come to terms with the fact that my intelligence had not cured my son, however. I also began to see that the people I met in Al-Anon had more wisdom than I did, and the reading I got at meetings made more sense than what I could figure out on my own. All of this was like having powers greater than myself.

· · · · ·

I know that I never would have made progress in recovery if I didn't let go of my ego and ask for help at my Families Anonymous meeting. I called people on the phone list and got literature each time I went to a meeting. I also took notes at each meeting about how the discussion related to things I needed to work on. My own way of working on things had gotten me nowhere. It was easy for me to take Step Two and Step Three because I knew that I needed to be restored to sanity. I couldn't do it by myself.

Parents can also struggle with the meaning of the word God in the Third Step. Three parents relate how they resolved this struggle:

I was suspicious of Step Two. At first, I thought it was about getting a God in church. I am not a big fan of organized religion because to me it is often about human beings screwing up God's message. I learned that Step Two and Step Three are not about having to go to church, though. They are all about realizing that you don't know everything, and you will be a lot better off if you realize that.

· · · · ·

For me, my God is a spiritual being, but it doesn't have to be this way. There is even a whole chapter in the Big Book *of AA about how atheists and agnostics can believe in the Third Step without believing in God.*

For me, however, I find that by praying and asking God to help me, I am able to receive guidance on what to do with my son and in a lot of other situations in my life.

· · · · ·

Step Two and Step Three actually increase my appreciation of going to church. The sanctuary is an inspiring place for prayer and meditation and special contact with God. Also, the Steps seem to help me focus more on what church is all about: the contact with a higher power and listening for God's will in your life. The Steps help me to not get so irritated with some of the other aspects of organized religion that I don't really think God cares about. The Twelve Steps have shown me the path to a much closer relationship with God.

Later recovery for adolescents

Once adolescents have accepted their powerlessness over drugs and alcohol in Step One and acknowledged that they need help in Steps Two and Three, they are ready for action. Step Three has actually prepared them for this action by asking them to relinquish control to a higher power. Their AA or NA sponsor becomes a form of this power as a facilitator or teacher for their later recovery.

In Step Four, adolescents are asked to do a written inventory of their lives, the good things they have done as well as the bad. They need to evaluate their character strengths and their character weaknesses. Step Four will help them validate their strengths and be honest about the weaknesses that might lead them back to drinking or using drugs. They will admit to these when they disclose them to their sponsor or another person of their choosing in Step Five.

These two inventory Steps are crucial to a successful recovery. They are designed to be painful because an honest inventory means admitting characteristics and behaviors that were often wished away by using alcohol or drugs. It will no longer be possible to bury these characteristics and behaviors or run away from them by using.

Parents often struggle with wishing that their children did not have to go through the pain with Steps Four and Five, particularly when they have changed so dramatically for the better as a result of early recovery. It is important for addicts/alcoholics to stay with their pain as they work through these Steps. The mother of an adolescent addict relates how important pain can be for continued recovery:

> *My son was so depressed when he was working on Step Four and Step Five. I talked about this with my parent-group counselor. She said that he had good reasons to be depressed because of the things he had done. She also said that staying in touch with this pain would help him stay sober.*
>
> *I learned that he should never forget the pain he caused himself or others as a result of his using. It is a form of enabling if I try to take the pain away. He needs it to be sober and drug-free.*

Further Step work will enhance the possibility that adolescents will continue with the recovery that results in productive, fulfilling lives. Outpatient and aftercare treatment programs will work hand in hand with reinforcing the importance of working on the Steps and doing whatever else is necessary for recovery to occur.

Adolescents working on recovery also need to substitute new behaviors for those that were part of their alcohol/drug-abusing lifestyle. The following list from an adolescent treatment program illustrates the choices adolescents need to make to be successful. The list is posted on large poster boards around the treatment center to help adolescents in outpatient treatment and aftercare focus on the actions they need to lead healthy, productive lives:

Positive Choices for Ongoing Recovery

> *Follow family rules—show respect.*
> *Have a sponsor.*
> *Have a home group.*
> *Go to meetings.*
> *Stay for fellowship after meetings.*
> *Sign up for coffee duty at your home group.*
> *Talk with people—get phone numbers.*
> *Read AA literature to work the Steps.*
> *Call people for rides.*
> *Call sponsor at minimum four to seven times a week.*
> *Call someone else in recovery four times a week.*
> *Have a daily routine to pray.*

Stay in dry places.
Stay with dry people.
Focus on yourself, not a relationship.
Talk about issues with supports.

This list can also be a good reminder to parents that it is their children who need to take responsibility for their own recovery; parents cannot do it for them.

Later recovery for parents

Once parents have accepted their powerlessness over drugs and alcohol—just like their teenagers—and acknowledged that they need help, they are ready for their own action steps to deepen their recovery.

The list of Positive Choices for Ongoing Recovery used for adolescents also applies to parents. For example, parents who ask others in their Al-Anon or Families Anonymous meetings to sponsor them will reap many benefits. They will have a mentor with the experience, strength, and hope that comes with more time in recovery. The parent of an adolescent addict discusses how a sponsor can help:

> *The counselor in my parent group encouraged us to get a sponsor at our Al-Anon or Families Anonymous meeting. She talked about how her own sponsor helped her. She said that a sponsor should be someone who seems to have solid recovery and is strong enough to not let us manipulate them. They wouldn't necessarily need to be someone who has an adolescent, because it isn't your child you will talk about, it is you.*

> *I approached a woman in my Al-Anon group and asked her if she would be my sponsor. I was scared that she would say no, but she said she was honored to be asked. She said that it would help her to deepen her own program by working with me.*

> *I have had her as a sponsor for several years now, and she has helped me a lot. She has encouraged me and been there for me when my son relapsed and ran away. She has also been tough on me about some of my weaknesses that I got in touch with by doing my Step Five with her. She helps me to focus on gratitude instead of self-pity and choosing forgiveness instead of staying in resentments. Negative characteristics only keep me in pain.*

She also gave me a plaque that says "Have a Good Day Unless You Have Made Other Plans."

She reminds me that I have choices. I don't have to be miserable.

When parents, like their adolescent children, call their sponsor four to seven times a week, and call their other new recovery friends at least four times a week, they begin to develop a close support system. This support system reduces the isolation that is felt by parents when their adolescents are abusing drugs and alcohol. The support can enrich lives in the beginning of recovery, and it takes on even greater meaning with time. A father who started Al-Anon when his son entered recovery relates how support has helped him and two other fathers:

My son is about to celebrate fifteen years of sobriety, which is a reminder of my anniversary as well. When I started in Al-Anon, I went to some groups that were specifically for men, and I met two other people like myself who were trying to detach from their alcoholics. We worked on the Steps together and, through this support, I started to have more serenity in my life.

We went out to dinner, just the three of us, once a month, and that has continued to this day. That's about 180 dinners where waitresses wondered who these three men were talking about feelings and how to have serenity!

We continue to encourage each other to not get on the personal roller coaster, which happens if we spend our time not working a recovery program. We have been there for each other as we have dealt with cancer in one man's son and a heroin relapse with another. We have also talked through work problems and issues around entering our 50s. These are my closest friends. I never would have had them if I hadn't reached out to find them in those early years of recovery.

When parents first enter recovery, they tend to focus more on their adolescent addicts/alcoholics than they do in later recovery. This is as a result of taking their Steps One, Two, and Three. Once that happens, recovery tends to focus more on quality of life issues regardless of how the alcoholic/addict is doing.

Parents who have taken their first three Steps share their stories of other things they are working on. In all cases, their adolescents are still struggling in treatment, but their parents have accepted that they are powerless over their children. They have moved on to focus on other aspects of their lives:

> When I first started recovery, I focused on how to detach from my son, but now I am working on how to detach from other people in my life who are doing destructive things. My son wasn't [the only one] hooking me; it was other people as well. It was like I was saying, "Here, come and abuse me. Come and take advantage of my good nature." My recovery has given me tools to be healthier and to set boundaries in my relationships.

· · · · ·

> I have moved along in my recovery, and I have started to work on how some of the patterns from my childhood still affect me. There are a lot of these patterns that helped me survive, but I don't need them any more. My parent-group counselor told me that I needed to do spring cleaning in my head, and she was right. My recovery program has given me the tools to accept my past and to forgive, but to not choose the old reactions.

· · · · ·

> I felt disposable when I was growing up. To make sure that people wouldn't throw me away, I became overly preoccupied with not screwing up. In my recovery, I am working on how I took over other people's responsibilities so they would like me. They took advantage of this, and I could not say no when they asked me to do things for them. I am trying to break this pattern. My recovery program helps me.

· · · · ·

> I first entered recovery to work on some issues related to my daughter, but now I am working on getting my own life going again. I had so preoccupied myself with her that I lost awareness of my own needs. I stopped reading because I couldn't concentrate, and I worried so much about the future that I couldn't even enjoy taking a walk and finding beauty in nature. I study my Al-Anon readings about living in the present and not projecting, and my sponsor helps me with sayings like, "I've had a lot of worries in my life, but most of them have never happened."

> I developed a lot of bad thinking habits when my daughter was using, and now I am trying to break them.

At the beginning of my recovery, I worked on accepting that I didn't have control over my son's drug addiction. I understood that no amount of lecturing or threatening was going to cure him, and that I had overused these out of my own fears as a way to control him.

Now I am working on how I do these same things to people at work. I am a supervisor with a lot of responsibilities to make sure things run the way they are supposed to, but I alienate a lot of people with my controlling, just like I alienated my family during the drug-using days. I need to humble myself to ask for help on this, but it is hard. I know that my recovery program will help me if I use it.

· · · · ·

My boss at work has told me that I have to work on how I am so focused on my job that I bottle all the stress inside. I don't exercise and I come across as intimidating and controlling.

I need to work on relaxing—easy does it—and not being such a controlling higher power with people. My recovery program helps me with this. I have to go right back to how my ego is getting in the way. I need to take Step One again, even though I have been in recovery for a while. It's not the alcoholic I am controlling now—it's other people.

Parents recovering in several programs

When parents are recovering from their own addiction in Alcoholics Anonymous or Narcotics Anonymous and bring their children for alcoholism/ addiction treatment, they have unique issues. They know the power of the disease. They have tried to control their children from following their path. They may also struggle with guilt because they were not able to see their teenager's addiction or alcoholism and find the magic words to cure them. The mother of an addict describes her frustration at being unable to control her daughter's alcoholism:

I was really depressed when we brought our daughter for treatment. I was reliving all the pain that I had when I was drinking at her age. Why hadn't I been able to save her from that?

I had been sober all of her life and had worked a strong recovery pro-gram in AA. She knew how drinking had led me down the wrong path. She had also heard how alcohol had destroyed the lives of her grandparents.

I had accepted Step One for my own drinking, but I needed Families Anonymous to help me with taking the Step again in another way. I had to work on how I did not have control over my daughter's illness, and that no lecture or reading was going to make her well. I couldn't cure her.

It amazed me that even though I knew a lot about the disease from my own personal experience, I was just like other parents in thinking I could make sure that addiction didn't happen with my own kids. In a way, my controlling was even worse. I was desperate to save them from the pain I went through.

Recovery values in your home

Parents often ask what they can do at home to support their adolescents in recovery. This will involve more than just saying that recovery is important. Teenagers, as well as younger children, listen more to what their parents do than to what they say. They are quick to see hypocrisy. When parents are able to practice recovery values and behaviors in their homes, they give a clear message that recovery is important. The recovering addict who has been sober since he was 16, and who gave the story of his surrender earlier in the chapter, relates to how important parents can be to ongoing recovery:

My parents entered into Twelve Step recovery immediately when I went to treatment and they were active in FA for years. They sponsored people and took leadership positions so that they could also help others. It made a big difference to me, because they weren't just labeling me as the family problem. They weren't just saying that they were going to sit at home and watch me; they were going to work on themselves, too. They even went without me for a week to Minnesota to the Hazelden family program so they could learn more about the disease.

Somehow, all of that made me feel supported. My parents really understood how powerful my disease was, and how they had to learn to deal with it. I was working hard, too, so we were all doing it together. Our family got even closer, and we are still very close today. I think that this support has really helped me stay straight these eighteen years.

Supporting recovery in your home is no guarantee that your child will not relapse, of course, just as parents cannot prevent their teenagers from becoming addicts/alcoholics. Even if adolescents ignore their parents' positive example, however, the parents can at least feel confident that they tried everything they could to help. In addition, parents will grow in their own recovery, and this will be especially helpful if their teenagers do not choose to get well.

It is important for parents to think about the recovery values in their home. The following list poses questions that are a starting point for thought and discussion:

- What values do I have? These will have an impact on my recovering adolescent.

- What is my commitment to using alcohol and drugs? Do my kids see that I drink to escape from stress? Do they watch me get defensive about my drinking? Does my drinking have harmful consequences on others and, also, on me?

- Does my lifestyle model recovery? Do I go to Twelve Step meetings just like I am asking my teenager to do? Do I read the literature and talk about what is helping me? Have I asked someone to be my sponsor? Do I call people in recovery to ask them for help?

- Do my lifestyle and conversation model the same kindness and respect for others which are core values in the recovery program my teenager is being asked to follow?

- Do I model that it is important to accept responsibility for your behavior like my teenager is being asked to do in recovery? Do I practice the same humility? Do I make amends for things I have done wrong?

- Do I show that I value my personal growth? Do I model that it is important to work on my imperfections?

Taking care of yourself

It is often difficult for parents to begin a recovery program, even when they know they are in pain as a result of what has been going on in their homes with their out-of-control addicts/alcoholics. Many parents who have shared their stories in earlier chapters have talked about wanting to be left alone. The desire for a long vacation is normal. On the other hand, parents who have entered their own recovery ha~~~~ Although they may not be alcoholics~~~~ inspired by the many promises of recovery ~~~~ Alcoholics Anonymous, particularly those found~~~~ Action. These promises are a reminder to all reco~~~~ parents, that there is hope if they work a program of re~~~~

Parents who did choose recovery will discuss the results of t~~~~ Chapter 11, Stories of Empowerment. The following promises a~~~~ Action in the Big Book. They are noted here for parents new to reco~~~~ are beginning their own journey:[4]

> We are going to know a new freedom and a new happiness. We will
> not regret the past nor wish to shut the door on it. We will comprehend the
> word serenity and we will know peace. No matter how far down the scale
> we have gone, we will see how our experience will benefit others. That
> feeling of uselessness and self-pity will disappear. We will lose interest in
> selfish things and gain interest in our fellows. Self-seeking will slip away.
> Our whole attitude and outlook upon life will change. Fear of people and
> of economic insecurity will leave us. We will intuitively know how to han-
> dle situations that used to baffle us. We will suddenly realize that God is
> doing for us what we could not do for ourselves.

Since these same promises are made to addicts working on recovery, they are another reminder of the similarities between the recovery programs of addicts/alcoholics and their families. Another similarity is the Serenity Prayer that was written by Reinhold Neibuhr as he struggled to survive in a German concentration camp. It is used today around the world in Twelve Step meetings and treatment programs as a reminder of the principles of recovery.

The Serenity Prayer[5]

God, grant me the serenity

to accept the things I cannot change,

courage to change the things I can,

and wisdom to know the difference.

The promises and the Serenity Prayer can provide inspiration and encouragement as parents face the challenges of working on their own recovery.

...ng Go

...ery, one of the first things they ...t Step challenges them to admit ...sult.

...s if they want to remove themselves from their person... ...le. On this ride, drug addicted/ alcoholic teenagers control their parent's steep descent, how long they stay down, and when they come up. Letting go means that parents don't buy their tickets in the first place.

Letting go is also important because holding on is a form of enabling. Alcoholics/addicts must experience the harmful consequences of their behaviors if they are going to get well. When parents do not let go, it is as if they are telling their teenagers that they want them to continue with their destructive lifestyle.

This chapter will discuss the difficulties with the letting-go process and, then, how letting go happens. This process usually starts with a focus on letting go of the addict/alcoholic's addiction and recovery. Once this happens, according to the promises of recovery, there is a new freedom, a new happiness. It is now possible to let go of other things. The mother of an addict describes how her life improved when she started to let go:

> When I first started my recovery, I worked on letting go of responsibility for what my son would have to work on for himself. Then I found that I was able to let go of other things. My life improved more than I ever could have imagined.
>
> I thought that the promises of recovery would never work for me. I believed in them, however, and I started to do the letting go work that

*would make them come true. Other parents can improve their lives, too.
They just need to believe that it is possible.*

Beginning the process of letting go

Before they can start the process of letting go, parents first need to take an inventory of how they release the stress that is bottled up inside. They will need this energy to work on letting go. Then parents need to review what they have learned about addiction and the codependent hooks that have led them to take responsibility for their teenager's substance abuse. They need to work on accepting that their teenagers are responsible for the work on their own recovery.

Creating positive energy

As described in Chapter 5, *Working on Your Feelings*, and Chapter 6, *Harmful Consequences from Normal Feelings*, it is normal to feel stressed and burned out when you are parents of addicts/alcoholics. If parents bring their adolescents to residential treatment, they often wish they could switch places and stay in the serene setting where residential programs usually operate. Why do their out-of-control teenagers get the benefit of this new environment? A mother relates how she needed time for herself:

> *When we brought our daughter to residential treatment, I looked out one of the large picture windows at a fawn that was nibbling on the grass. It was a beautiful fall day and the trees had started to blaze with color. Everything was so serene. I wished that we could send my daughter home, and my husband and I could move in. We needed a vacation!*
>
> *I also found myself resenting my daughter because she was coming to this beautiful place. She was the one that had made our life so miserable. We needed the time out. What about our needs?*
>
> *It seemed so unfair. She was going to watch deer nibbling on the grass while her father and I were going to be at home when her drug-using friends called. We were going to have to watch these so-called friends come to our door. We were going to have to stand there and ask them to leave. We were going to be the ones to explain to people at church or in the grocery store where our daughter was.*

We were also being told that we had to drive back to the treatment site three times a week and to Families Anonymous meetings, and that we would need to start working on our own recovery. Where were we supposed to get the energy for all this?

It is often difficult to have the motivation to create energy when you are feeling exhausted and burned out from activities and resentments. Parents who have a daily exercise program know that exercise creates energy, however, even when they feel exhausted. This is because sitting around and stressing out—without the advantage of blood cells getting new oxygen—makes you feel even more tired than you actually are. In addition, physical exercise helps free negative emotional energy that is trapped inside your body, the energy that leads you to be edgy and defensive. This trapped energy can also lead to the angry outbursts that parents regret and wish they could undo. The mother of an addict describes how exercise helped her:

I couldn't believe how much better I felt when my parent-group counselor recommended exercise. I had a treadmill in my bedroom that I hadn't used for almost a year, and I started running on it every day as soon as I got home from work and changed my clothes. It was only a fifteen-minute workout to start with, but it made me feel better about myself and I was much less defensive with my kids.

A daily exercise program of even a brisk fifteen-minute walk is going to be helpful in doing the work of letting go in recovery. There are a variety of other healthy stress-reduction techniques as well, and parents will need to find what works for them. Appendix A, *Resources,* lists *The Relaxation Response* by Herbert Benson, which will help with ideas.

Accepting the three Cs

When parents begin the letting-go process, they also need to review what they have learned about addiction. The Serenity Prayer challenges parents "To accept the things [they] cannot change," and "To have the courage to change the things [they] can." It is not possible for parents to change the fact that their adolescents are addicts or alcoholics. On the other hand, it is possible to change how to deal with them.

To summarize points made in previous chapters:

- Addiction involves a love relationship with alcohol and drugs.

- No matter how bad or good parents have been, they do not cause their children's addiction.

- Parents cannot cure, nor can they control, whether their children choose recovery.

Parents are always working on accepting the three Cs: they did not *cause*, they cannot *control*, and they cannot *cure* their children's addiction/alcoholism. The mother of an addict/alcoholic in his early 30s describes how working on herself has made it possible to accept the power of her son's disease:

> *Our son went to treatment when he was 17. He even graduated from his highly respected treatment program after seven months of residential treatment.*
>
> *Many of the kids who graduated from that program when we were there have remained sober and have seventeen or eighteen years of sobriety. Our son has had a difficult time of it, however. We tried every way we could to support him without being enablers and got wonderful help from friends in Families Anonymous. We worked on accepting the power of his disease and [on the fact] that he was the one who had to take responsibility for his recovery. It was hard for us because we wanted to fix him. We wanted to make sure that he would have a happy future. We learned through trying, however, that we couldn't control his life the way we wanted to.*
>
> *Our son says that he loves us, and that he is proud of how we don't get hooked by him. He looks at us with his big blue eyes, and it is so easy to remember when he was small enough for his little bottom to fit in the pocket of my elbow. We have moved on, and our life is definitely not on hold, but we love our son, and it is hard to watch him destroy himself. It's all so sad.*
>
> *We are happy that we have worked on ourselves, however. You never know what your addict is going to choose.*

Being responsible to, and not for, your children

Part of accepting that you cannot control and you cannot cure your addict/ alcoholic teenagers is accepting that you are responsible to them, but not for them. The distinction between "to" and "for" can be difficult for parents to grasp. Doing so is very important to letting go, however.

Parents have a history of struggling with the word "responsibility." They often use the word when they first discuss whether or not they are ready to have children. Are they ready for this new responsibility? Later, the word is used to describe greater or lesser responsibility with whatever is happening in their children's lives. Parents may also hear the word when others tell them that they are responsible for paying for a window their child has broken. They hear from teachers that they will be responsible for monitoring their children's homework.

Table 9-1 describes the difference between being responsible for others and being responsible to others.

Table 9-1. Responsibility

	Responsible for Others	**Responsible to Others**
I am concerned with:	Answers	Empowering
	Fixing	Being compassionate
	Controlling	Being respectful
I feel:	Tired	Energized
	Anxious	Calm
	Put upon	Peaceful
	Used	Supported by others
	Depressed	Serene
	Self-neglectful	Whole
I do:	Minimize	Empathize
	Protect	Confront
	Deny	Accept
	Rescue	Let go

The key words in this figure are the words "to" and "for." Even when their children are not addicts/alcoholics, parents have trouble with these words and what they mean in terms of misplaced responsibility. It is easy to take responsibility for their children's behaviors. For example, when parents take responsibility "for" their children, they end up doing the homework that their children have put off. They also drive their children to school after they choose to sleep an extra ten minutes and miss the bus.

These parental rescuing behaviors—doing for—may include a lecture implying that this is the last time the parents will "help" them, but it usually isn't.

Children learn to count on being helped, which amounts to being rescued. They also learn they do not really need to be responsible for procrastinating, oversleeping, or whatever else has a potential negative consequence. They do not have to worry and, thereby, take more responsibility for themselves. Someone will bail them out.

Parents can often feel used, depressed, and tired when they take responsibility for their children's behaviors. On the other hand, this can be justified by believing that the overall goal is worth it: children will be happy; they will have better grades, a perfect, on-time attendance record, the best science project, or whatever else parents have taken responsibility for. In fact, parents are working harder for these goals than their children are. No wonder parents feel tired. In addition, their children have not really learned how to manage their time and their lives by following through on their own and seeing the results of their efforts.

Complications with abuse and addiction

The problem of taking on some of your children's responsibilities is compounded when they become substance-abusing teenagers. As part of the normal family response to substance abuse discussed in Chapter 1, *Use, Abuse, and Dependency,* parents have often taken over responsibilities for their drug-abusing, addict/alcoholic adolescents as well as for their feelings, their behaviors, and the consequences of their drug/alcohol abuse. Reasons for this are in Chapter 6, where codependency, enabling, and parenting traps are discussed. It often happens that parents find themselves giving in to their teenagers more than they want to, feeling sorry for them, and overlooking their irresponsible behaviors. They lend money to their teenagers, for example, even though there is a history that this money does not get paid back. It also happens many drug-abusing, addicted adolescents' parents are so intimidated by their anger that their teenagers have virtually taken over control of the family; there are no rules that parents can enforce.

Two mothers of addicts discuss how shifts in responsibility happened when their adolescents were abusing drugs:

> *I told my son that he would have consequences if he stayed out late or didn't clean his room, or if he didn't improve his grades. He got so sarcastic and defiant when I talked about consequences, however, that I never followed up with action. He said that I was too strict and that he had poor teachers. I felt responsible to get him out of his mess by helping*

him more, so I started to just ignore his problems and made excuses for him. I told his teachers how I thought they needed to teach, and I worked on being a more modern parent that didn't have rules.

I actually thought that I was somehow responsible for what he was doing. I had to figure out solutions. I felt depressed and anxious, however, because the problems only got worse. Then I blamed myself because somehow I wasn't being a good enough parent. If I were, things wouldn't be falling apart so much.

· · · · ·

My daughter was not having the kind of teenage life that I had hoped she would have, because she started getting into trouble. Then she got pregnant at 15, and 9 months later we were taking care of her baby at home.

She helped with the baby the first few months, but when she went back to high school, she wanted to hang out with her friends and not be at home. After dinner, for example, she didn't want to give the baby his bath and put him to bed, she wanted to go out.

I wanted her to have the normal teenage life, so I started taking over responsibilities with my grandchild. It got to the point that he didn't even want to be with his mother anymore. I felt guilty asking her to help; then my grandson would cry since I wasn't taking care of him.

I felt that I was responsible for my daughter to have a happy life. She was only 16. I wanted her to be normal. I started feeling used, but then I would feel guilty that I wasn't content. My daughter kept telling me that she needed more freedom. I felt that if I were a good mother, I would do everything to help her have this freedom. When other family members said that she should take more responsibility for her baby, I made excuses for her. I tried to fix everything so she looked more responsible than she really was.

We found out later that she had a secret life all this time, and I made it easier for her. I had no idea that she was partying with her friends and that she was using drugs like cocaine. She knew that I wanted her to be happy, and she took advantage of this. Now I am working on not enabling her.

When adolescents first enter recovery, it is easy for the shifts in responsibility to happen because parents are not often strong enough in their own programs. Several fathers describe how their addict/alcoholic teenagers pulled them in and what they had to do:

> It was so hard for me to watch my daughter have pain. She felt lonely that she had to do all these things in recovery. I wasn't very strong myself, and I went right back to feeling that I had to make her happy. I took responsibility for making sure that she wasn't sad, as if it was something I had to work on. I even lied to her outpatient counselor and said that she went to more AA meetings than she really did. She said she felt depressed when she went to those meetings since she didn't know anybody. I didn't want her to feel unhappy by lying, so I decided to cover for her.
>
> This is exactly what I did in the using days when I would tell her school that she had a cold when she really had a hangover. I also lied about some vandalism she did in the community when I told the police that she was at home with her parents.
>
> I obviously have to work on how I take over responsibility for her to look good. She needs to put more energy into this than I do. I have taught her that she doesn't really have to work hard at it, however. She thinks that I will do it for her. I am working on how I rescue her.

· · · · ·

> I thought that the staff at our outpatient program was too tough on our son when they said that he was supposed to be responsible for getting rides to and from AA meetings. They said that members of Alcoholics Anonymous and Narcotics Anonymous do this transportation thing as part of working their own programs. Driving with them would be good for my son because they would [form a] fellowship and talk about the meeting.
>
> My son said that he felt uncomfortable asking for rides, so I drove him myself. I even went into the meetings with him. We agreed that we wouldn't tell his counselor, however. He didn't really understand my son anyway, or so I thought. I was tired from those late nights, but I had to go with him to make sure he stayed straight.
>
> What I found out, of course, is that my son was using drugs all that time, and he was only going to AA meetings to keep his counselor off his

back. He didn't want to drive with AA people because he was afraid they would discover his secret.

I believed him when he said that I was helping him stay straight. I liked it when he said that because I could take some credit for his recovery. Now I see that I was right back to trying to fix things. It was just like the old using days when I would bail him out of trouble.

When parents take responsibility for their teenagers' behaviors, whether it's a missed bus, a drug addiction, or the process of recovery, they have the negative consequences of feeling tired, anxious, and depressed. They are often fearful that if they don't keep up with these behaviors, their teenagers' lives will fall apart.

Unfortunately, however, their adolescents are not experiencing negative consequences for their behaviors. They have denial about the fact that procrastinating leads to problems or they rationalize that they can lie to their treatment counselors because their parents already do this. Just like in the drug-using days, lying is permissible.

Choosing positive behaviors

On the other hand, when parents let themselves be responsible to, rather than for, their adolescents' behaviors, they can encourage them when they do get up on time, but let them walk or take other forms of transportation than the family car when they don't. They can encourage their children to plan their time so they can complete their homework, but let them experience the harmful consequences when they do not. They can encourage them to follow through with their treatment assignments, but not lie for them when they do not.

Parents can also choose to use what they have learned about addiction. If addict/alcoholics do not take responsibility for the work in their recovery, despite their loneliness or other pain, they will not get well. Parents must accept that being responsible for their adolescents, and not letting go, will cripple them.

Stage one: Letting go

When parents are responsible to their alcoholic/addict teenagers and let go, they support their teenagers' recovery as well as their own. Parents feel confused about the letting go process at the beginning, however. They wonder if it means they no longer love their adolescents. They struggle with feeling that letting go means they no longer care about them, and they sometimes think that letting go means they are bad parents. The mother of an addict describes how letting go is a strong form of parental love:

> I was confused about letting go until I realized that it is actually the strongest form of parental love. I can really help my children grow when they take responsibility for themselves.
>
> This kind of love is even more difficult than giving in to my children. I have a history of spoiling them by satisfying their every desire, and cleaning up all of their mistakes. We know that spoiled children lead to spoiled adults. Letting go helps to create mature, responsible children who grow to be mature, responsible adults. Isn't this what every parent wants?

The following list of letting go behaviors is widely circulated in Al-Anon and Families Anonymous meetings. The principles describe what parents need to do to encourage their children's maturity and recovery:

> To let go…
>
> Does not mean to stop caring, it means I can't do it for someone else.
>
> Is not to cut myself off, it's the realization that I can't control another.
>
> Is not to enable, but to allow learning from natural consequences.
>
> Is to admit powerlessness, which means that the outcome is not in my hands.
>
> Is not to try to change or blame another, it's to make the most of myself.
>
> Is not to care for, but to care about.
>
> Is not to fix, but to be supportive.
>
> Is not to judge, but to allow another to be a human being.
>
> Is not to be in the middle arranging all the outcomes, but to allow others to affect their destinies.

Is not to be protective, it's to permit another to face reality.

Is not to deny, but to accept.

Is not to nag, scold or argue, but, instead, to search out my own shortcomings and correct them.

Is not to adjust everything to my own desires, but to take each day as it comes and cherish myself in it.

Is not to criticize or regulate anybody, but to try to become what I dream I can be.

Is not to regret the past, but to grow and live for the future.

Is to fear less, and love more.

Parents' early struggles with letting go

Parents who are in recovery and who try to practice the principles of Al-Anon, Nar-Anon, or Families Anonymous usually know that letting go is important, but they struggle with what the principles mean. They share the following stories of what they struggled with in the early stages of recovery and how they changed:

Early in my recovery, people said that I needed to learn acceptance of my daughter's addiction and that the only way that she would be able to have recovery was to see the consequences of her choices.

It seems to me that what I was supposed to do was cruel; sort of like a mother robin pushing her baby off the roof when all it can do is crash on the cement below. My parent-group counselor said that if I really understood what addiction was, and accepted that my daughter is an addict, I would know that I couldn't cure her.

This is so hard for me. It is really impossible for me to feel powerless over anything, particularly something bad that is threatening my daughter. Addiction threatens her life. Letting go was one of the hardest things I ever had to do. I really needed my Families Anonymous meetings to help me.

• • • • •

My wife and I had a lot of fears about our son going back to school after he was in treatment. Some people recommend that he have home schooling, but he is 17 and has a lot of energy, so what would he have done the rest of the day?

We can't really organize his life for him, but we felt responsible to do this. We weren't strong enough in our own recovery, so it was easy to go back to the old enabling. We had learned how important it was to help addicts be responsible for their own recovery. This was really hard, though. Letting go goes against every instinct parents have to protect their children. It is overwhelming to realize that we can't.

· · · · ·

We were so afraid of our daughter going back to her using friends after treatment. She seemed to have washed her hands of them, but it was at the point that she had no friends, none. Our fear was that the only friends that would accept her back were her user friends.

Our Al-Anon friends said that she needed to take responsibility for finding new friends in recovery by going to AA meetings. They said that she needed to accept responsibility to get rides to meetings. We had to let go of the fear that she was going to relapse with these people. If she did, that was her consequence, not ours.

Parents whose adolescents have a dual-diagnosis have additional struggles with letting go. Two parents describe these struggles and how they work on themselves:

One of the big things I have had to work on is how to let go around my daughter's dual-diagnosis issues. We found out when she had her assessment that not only is she an addict, she is also manic-depressive. She is now on lithium in addition to being in recovery for cocaine and marijuana addiction.

On the one hand, I am relieved. She has had mood swings that were not normal since she was a little girl. Now we know what they were all about. I knew in third grade that something was wrong with her. I have this fantasy that now she will be happy.

On the other hand, I am really scared. I want to help her, but I don't want to let her out of my sight. I have so much fear about the dose of lithium because it has to be leveled out. I am also afraid that she won't take her medication. If she abuses her medication, this could trigger a relapse

on cocaine as well. Then I am afraid that she won't work a recovery pro-
gram at all. She will be right back on the streets.

She has to be responsible for so much, and I continue to struggle with
letting go. It has really helped that I have some close friends that I met at
Families Anonymous. They have helped me through the rough times.

· · · · ·

My son has the dual-diagnosis of attention deficit disorder and
cocaine addiction. He's on medication and I am so grateful that he has a
psychiatrist that understands addiction and recovery.

I panic that my son will lose his sobriety if he doesn't get it together.
Then I organize his life for him. He's almost 18. I need to let go so he can
take more responsibility for these things, but it drives me nuts to hold my
tongue so much. It's almost like I need to stuff a big wad of cotton in my
mouth to help me be quiet. This is one of the hardest things I have ever
done. My Families Anonymous program has really helped me.

Caring about, and not for, your children

Twelve Step recovery helps parents work on resolving many of the difficulties of letting go. Parents learn to stay in the present, for example, to live one
day at a time and not project into the future. Recovery also helps parents
work on substituting faith for fear and to realize that practicing a new form
of love is the one thing they can do to help their addict/alcoholic. Recovery
helps them care about their teenagers, but not care for them. A father who
has been in Families Anonymous for several years describes how caring
about, and not for, has given him a new relationship with his son:

What I have learned in my own recovery is how to respect and love
my son on even deeper levels by caring about him rather than for him.
This gives him the dignity of making his own choices and dealing with his
own consequences. I can care about him, but not get in his way.

I have learned how to have boundaries so he can't take advantage of
me, and I have also learned how to detach so he feels the consequences of
his behavior. I have come to love him on a healthier level because the love
doesn't involve trying to make him into the person I want him to be. I
think he feels this respect.

The interesting thing is that he has more energy to set high goals for himself because these are his goals, not mine. I think that our story is an example of how when you help yourself, you are also helping your kids. When I let go, a lot of good things happened for my son and me.

Now I can care about things that are going on his life. I can be there to assist him if I have something he needs help with, but I can't solve his problems. I can't make things okay with the police department. I can't rescue him by coming up with bail money if he gets in trouble. I can't control his addiction, or if he is drinking or using drugs. He has to be responsible to get up on time, and do what he has to do.

Through my own recovery, I can now say to my son that I love you, but I hate what you are doing. There is such freedom in that love, for both my son and me.

Stage two: Letting go

Parents often begin their letting go process by focusing on their relationship with their addict/alcoholic teenagers. It quickly becomes apparent that letting go principles apply to other relationships in their lives.

Letting go of a spouse or co-parent

When adolescents are abusing drugs and alcohol, it is normal for them to manipulate their parents to get what they want. As described in Chapter 7, *Communication and Relationships*, parents often take on opposite roles in the family to keep the peace. One is the Super Parent and the other is the Prosecutor. Like pulling two ends of taffy, the roles pull away from each other and the relationship falls on the floor. These patterns of behavior will continue unless there is effort to change them. The father of an addict shares how he and his wife had to work on their relationship:

My wife and I fought a lot during our daughter's use, and it was a relief to have her enter residential treatment. We thought that all our problems would be over by having her out of the house.

But then we fought about our daughter not obeying the rules of the treatment program. It really bothered me that she couldn't obey rules, and I got very upset about it.

*After that, we started fighting about how much to talk in our treat-
ment groups. My wife is more outspoken about everything. I find it more
difficult to share. We would fight about that, because we wanted the other
person to change. I wasn't comfortable doing it her way. I resented how
she was pushing me. She resented that I wasn't more like her.*

*Our partnership had the same problems we had when our daughter
was at home. This helped us to see that we had things to work on for ourselves. We have different styles in the way we deal with stress and how we
express ourselves. We needed to work on accepting those in each other at
the same time we were working on co-parenting. There were some old
patterns we had to let go of with each other before we started to get well.*

Parents also need to let go of the co-parent because as long as they do not,
they are not working on themselves. Two parents describe how they focused
on their spouse and what they needed to do to change:

*When we first started treatment with our daughter, she was the rea-
son we were there. For the first three weeks in every group, however, all I
could think about was my husband. There were a lot of things bottled up
inside me from everything we had been through with our daughter. I had
to work on letting those go before I could even listen for what I needed to
work on.*

*I am glad that I worked on letting go of my husband, however. I had
a lot of my own stuff. If I had kept the focus on him, I never would have
made the positive changes that have helped me grow.*

· · · · ·

*When my wife and I started in the parent group at our son's treat-
ment program, I was so glad that my wife was there. She had been such
an enabler of our son, and it would drive me crazy how she would give in
to him.*

*I made sure that I would sit next to my wife in the parent group so I
could nudge her when the counselor would say things that related to her.
When we went on breaks, I would rehash what we had already heard to
make sure she understood it.*

*I was sure that I would get better if she changed. I knew that I lost
my temper more than I should and that I was spending too much time*

with my buddies playing golf, but if and when my wife got better, I would stop these behaviors. I would have no desire to get mad, and I would want to be at home to help out. Everything negative that I was doing was my wife's fault.

Our parent counselor overheard one of my lectures to my wife one week when we were on a break. I could tell that she was looking at me with one of those all-knowing expressions. She smiled as if she was glad that I was being so direct with my wife about how she had made mistakes in raising our son. I was really happy and very smug: the counselor was on my side. My wife was sick and needed help! I had been the perfect parent all along!

When we started the group again, the counselor looked right at me. She said that she wanted us to write down the name of our spouse or co-parent because we were going to put them in a box. She held up the box and said that once we had done that, we were going to put the lid on. I smiled to myself. Now we were now being given the freedom to say on paper that this spouse had been the source of all the problems. How clever that we were putting them in a box. I was still mad at my wife because my advice didn't seem to be changing her. I liked the idea of stuffing her in a box!

What happened next really surprised me, however. The parent-group counselor said that we were putting the names in the box because we needed to let go of the need to control them. We were turning them over to their Higher Power, and that's why we were putting the lid on. As long as we were focusing on our spouse or co-parent, we were not focusing on ourselves. She said that everyone in the room had something that they needed to work on. Taking the other person's inventory was enough to start with; that showed arrogance.

She also said that when we think that all of our problems will be over when the other person changes, we are in trouble. We think we are perfect, and it is up to others to make us happy. She asked us to think about how that comes across to others. She reminded us that other people might not want to change. We can only change ourselves.

I have since realized that I had a lot of arrogant thinking to work on. I will never forget that day with the box. The tables got turned on me, but it was the beginning of looking at myself and starting to grow.

Adolescent addicts/alcoholics will continue to try to manipulate their parents with old behaviors when they are in early recovery. They do not yet have strong enough recovery behaviors. If parents allow these manipulations, they are right back to the enabling, codependent behaviors they are trying to undo. Whether parents are married or divorced, they need to work together if recovery is going to progress with their teenagers. They also need to work on letting go of issues so they can work on themselves. The focus needs to be on themselves, not others.

Letting go in other relationships

When parents make progress in letting go of their adolescents' choices, they see how they can improve their relationships with others. The codependency patterns in a family discussed in Chapter 6 also relate to how parents get hooked with friends and colleagues at work. Recovery helps undo these interactions. Two mothers share stories about how letting go and recovery helped them with others:

> When my daughter was in treatment, I learned a lot about how I took over responsibilities for her when she pushed the "feel sorry for me" button. I worked hard on letting go. I learned how to say no to her.
>
> I started to realize that I let people at work take advantage of me, too. I wanted everyone to like me, the same trap that I got into with my daughter. I became aware of the fact that I could work an Al-Anon program at work, too, even when I wasn't with alcoholics.

· · · · ·

> When my son came to treatment, I worked hard on letting go of rescuing patterns that were enabling him and leaving me feeling burned out. People were coming to me with their problems, but they were expecting me to solve them. I felt responsible to help them. It was my job to get them out of their misery and whatever was causing it.
>
> I started to get people off my responsibility list. I realized that I had friends who lived by want, want, want. I had actually taught them to be this way with me. They really weren't there for my needs. I had to realize that I had taught them that I didn't have any needs since I never asked for help.
>
> I started to look at how I was giving in relationships, but I wasn't getting anything back in return. I was even choosing friends that didn't have

much to give. I liked how they were dependent on me. I started to see how I was setting up my own loneliness by not having healthier friends.

I had to start letting go of people in my life that were monkeys on my back. They were weighing me down. I needed to do this so I could be healthier myself. It wasn't my job to be responsible for everyone. There was no "me" left with all that. I had to get a "me" back in order to make something out of myself.

A father also relates how his recovery program helped him in other relationships:

When we first started to get help for our son, I worked on how to not take responsibility for what he was doing. This was hard. I was embarrassed about his vandalism in the community and that we were getting calls from the police. One of the worst days was when a police car actually came to our house and parked in my driveway. What would the neighbors think of that?

I was covering up for my son more than I knew was right, but I didn't want people to think that we were unfit parents. People are so quick to judge if kids have problems and do destructive things. I judged other parents myself.

I had to let go of what the neighbors thought. I was letting my fears of their judgments lead me to lying for my son. I was not only enabling him, but I was falling into the trap of changing my own values in order for him to like me. I learned that lying for him only taught him that when he lied himself, that was okay, too.

Then I looked at how I was taking responsibility for all the people I was supervising at work. I wanted my department to look good. When my employees messed up, I covered it up. I didn't want people to think that I had made hiring mistakes. If I were really a good supervisor, we would have perfect employees. I covered up for mistakes and even lied about them. I never fired anyone. Doing so would be to admit that I hadn't done my own job right.

Needless to say, my employees took advantage of this. Also, it was clear to outsiders that some people who worked under me were not right for the job, but I didn't listen to them. There was even one experience where I promoted someone I had gotten negative feedback about. I was so intent on proving that I had done the right thing in hiring this person. The organization was now suffering because of my sick thinking.

I had to work on not letting my feelings about myself get so enmeshed with the performance of others. I had to separate myself from feeling responsible for how others perform. I had to let go of feeling responsible for their consequences. I had to work on letting go the people under my supervision who were not right for the job.

I am still working on this, but I am so grateful that I understand how my codependency has affected me in my family as well as in my work life. When we first came to treatment, I had no idea that it could help me in other aspects of my life.

Letting go of the past

When parents work on their recovery, they also realize that they can use their program to let go of the past. Several mothers share how their lives improved by letting go:

I did a lot of work in my recovery on how I held on to some painful feelings that related to being adopted. I grew up feeling discarded. I had to make sure people liked me so they wouldn't throw me away.

Some other things happened, too, where people in my life left. I thought these things were just more of the same. This is what my life was going to be like.

This kind of thinking really messed me up with being a parent and with just about every relationship in my life. I let people take advantage of me and abuse me. I felt that I was responsible for everyone's happiness. I was terrified that they would throw me away if I didn't please them.

I really worked on accepting that my biological parents did the best they could in giving me up. They were just teenagers. I was just an infant. They didn't really know me anyway.

I accepted that all the situations in my life where I felt discarded were just that, situations. The circumstances led to me being discarded. They were not because of something I had done. I also worked on accepting that *people in my past had their own problems that were, and are, outside of my control, then and now. I had to work on praying for them, and turning them over to their Higher Power. My resentments about them were only ruining my peace of mind, not theirs.*

It was so important for me to let go of my past. I couldn't have done this without the help of my recovery program. I am happier today than I would have ever thought possible.

· · · · ·

I had a lot of recovery work to do to let go of my childhood. My mother was an alcoholic, and she married a whole lot of alcoholics. My biological father was mentally ill. None of the adults who raised me had made it. This meant that I was damaged. I didn't have any positive genes to give me strength.

When I had my own failed marriage, this only confirmed to me that I was a loser. I was a very weak mother because I couldn't trust my own instincts. My kids took advantage of me, and I felt that I deserved this. When our son came to treatment for cocaine addiction, I was so depressed and detached. I thought that his addiction was my fault.

We started our treatment, but all I could do was cry. I started to get well in my parent group when the counselor just let me sit there with a box of tissue. There was no pressure to talk. She even played music, and it helped me to get more in touch with my pain. She kept encouraging me to get the pain out. It felt so safe to cry.

Then she told me how strong I was that I had survived my childhood. I had never thought of myself as strong, so that was new. I even remember looking at myself in the mirror one day. I looked different, somehow. As I look back, that was a turning point. I was starting to see that I had strengths inside; if I could only get these strengths out, I could substitute them for all the stuff that was keeping me weak.

My recovery went on from there, and I had a lot of work to do. I had to let go of thinking about myself as damaged. I began to appreciate my strengths. I did a lot of reading from a list of books I got from my parent-group counselor. I especially loved an author who calls herself SARK, because she really helped me celebrate myself. I even went out and bought fingerpaints. I let myself be a kid who is creative, just like SARK recommended. I was discovering that I had a joyful side, and that surprised me, too.

I also had some individual therapy and kept going to my Families Anonymous meetings. People cared about me there. They really encouraged me.

My parent-group counselor kept telling me that growing is like doing spring-cleaning in your head. I was really excited with all the things I was sweeping out. I kept thinking about all the trash bags I was piling up.

Taking care of yourself

Working on letting go can be both scary and exciting. Parents who do the work find that they are able to make major changes in the way they relate to their past, their addict/alcoholic teenagers, and others in their lives.

Parents who think they are worth recovery get energized to keep going. Stories in this chapter illustrate that the hard work is worth it. Remember the story of the little engine that could. You can because you think you can. It is also helpful to remember these words of an anonymous prayer passed around at Al-Anon meetings:

The Codependent's Serenity Prayer

God, grant me the serenity

To accept the people I cannot change,

The courage to change the person I can,

And the wisdom to know that that person is me.

CHAPTER 10

Providing Natural Consequences

What you live with, you learn.

—Anonymous

DRUG AND ALCOHOL ABUSERS and addicts/alcoholics need to experience the natural consequences of their use if they are going to reverse course and end their self-destructive lifestyles. When parents begin to realize that they are only getting in the way when they rescue their teenagers, they are on the way to helping them. This is part of the work of letting go.

This chapter will explain natural consequences, help you understand how to provide them, and discuss what children and teenagers learn when natural consequences are given. Examples will show how these consequences can be applied to alcoholics/addicts by letting them know in advance what is expected of them. Parents who have been working on recovery programs will illustrate how providing natural consequences has benefited them and their families. Lastly, an alcoholic/addict in recovery for almost twenty years will describe the impact of consequences on her recovery.

Raising responsible children

Many have written about the challenges of raising responsible children. The best insights often come from professionals who treat those who are irresponsible. These professionals have to help individuals be motivated to reverse their irresponsible, non-productive behaviors.

In the mid-1960s, psychiatrist William Glasser, MD, writing about patients in psychotherapy in his book *Reality Therapy*, stated that:

> *Therapy will be successful when patients are able to give up denying the world and recognize that reality not only exists, but they must fulfill their needs within its framework.*[1]

Glasser based his theories on his work with patients who were trying to become more responsible. According to his wife, Naomi, in her book of case studies, *Control Theory in the Practice of Reality Therapy*:

> *Glasser was dissatisfied with what he had been taught, especially the idea that people with psychological problems are not responsible for their behavior.*[2]

Glasser was somewhat revolutionary in the more Freudian psychiatric circles of the time because he did not think that years of analysis were necessary for patients to become more responsible and get well. He said that therapy should be focused on having patients look at the reality of their lives in terms of what they want, and what they are doing to get what they want. They need to ask themselves if what they are doing is working. If not, what should they do differently? He also wrote that patients need to look at their needs and adjust their needs to fit the reality of their world.

In developing and refining his theories in the early 1960s, Glasser applied them to one of the most difficult of populations, severely delinquent adolescents. Their behaviors were similar to those of the alcoholics/addicts who are the focus of this book. His work with adolescent girls at the Ventura School in California is described in detail in *Reality Therapy* and shows how consistent warmth and discipline—working together—can help even the most irresponsible adolescents become more responsible.

Glasser has been a prolific writer and teacher along with his wife, Naomi, and his colleague, Robert E. Wubbolding. His theories are widely accepted today, and they are often quoted when the subjects of providing natural consequences and raising responsible children are discussed.

Glasser also relates his theories to institutions for children, such as schools. He describes how adults can help children look at the consequences of their behaviors, whether their behaviors are working, and what they need to do to change. His books *Schools Without Failure* and *Quality Schools* illustrate how nurturing environments that provide logical, natural consequences can both motivate children toward acceptable behaviors and help them grow to be mature adults.

Glasser's principles can also be applied at home. Parents interested in learning more about his theories and how to apply them will find the books and authors discussed here listed in Appendix A, *Resources*.

The importance of natural consequences

It is especially important for adolescent drug/alcohol abusers and addicts/alcoholics to experience natural consequences, but all children need to experience them to become mature, responsible adults. This is because the mature adult world operates on the premise that behaviors do have consequences. To be mature means that you recognize this reality and plan accordingly.

Natural consequences follow the rules of nature and physics: you are hungry if you do not eat, cold if you do not dress warmly, or burned if you touch fire. These are consequences parents usually impress upon their young children.

Logical consequences are based on social order and are not always instinctive. For example, if a young child is having a tantrum, a logical consequence is for the parent to leave the room. The child learns that being out of control causes people to move away from him. He learns that tantrums don't work to get what he wants.

Without realizing it, however, parents also teach consequences they may not have intended—such as, cry long enough, and I will read you an extra bedtime story; complain loud enough, and you won't have to do your chores; yell at me, and I will let you do whatever you want. Parents need to be careful what they are teaching. Consider the following:

- Natural and logical consequences encourage children to be responsible for their own behavior. Natural consequences are those that permit children to learn from the natural order of the physical world. (Example: don't eat, and you will be hungry.)

- Logical consequences are those that permit children to learn from the reality of the social order (i.e., tell lies, and people won't trust you).

- For consequences to be effective, they need to make sense to children.

- The purpose of using natural and logical consequences is to motivate children to make responsible decisions, not to force submission.

- Consequences are effective only if you avoid having the hidden motives of winning and controlling.

- Parents must work together in presenting and following through with consequences.

The last point is very important. Even if they are divorced, parents need to present a united front regarding consequences. Children manipulate around consequences, and parents do not want to reinforce these manipulations. The mother of an addict shares lessons she and her husband regret:

> *Without realizing it, my husband and I were teaching our daughter that if she used charm and self-pity, she didn't have to face the reality of her consequences. This was because one or the other of us would give in when we should have been firm. We allowed our daughter to manipulate us. We were not teaching her mature behaviors.*

Punishment and natural consequences

Parents often confuse providing consequences with being in control of their children. Children are quick to lose respect for their parents when consequences are not logical and are used with intimidation and power to inspire fear. Also, children do not learn respect for rules from these consequences. A father describes how he learned to distrust authority:

> *I grew up with an alcoholic father who would go on rage attacks and hit me with his shaving belt or send me out in our two-acre yard to pick dandelions all afternoon. He would say that I did something or other, but it was all so arbitrary I had no idea why I was being punished. He just wanted power.*
>
> *I was certainly afraid of him, but I had no respect for him, and he didn't really teach me about logical, natural consequences. What I learned was to distrust authority, and I had trouble with rebellion later in life. I had no concept that authority figures could be fair, and my sense of consequences from misbehavior was way out of whack. The world was just unfair and illogical.*

Children and teens may perceive any unpleasant consequence for their behavior as punishment, but it is important to distinguish between punitive consequences decided at the will of a parent and undesirable consequences that flow logically from the behavior of the child or teen.

There are many differences between punishment and natural, logical consequences:

- Punishment expresses the power of personal authority. Logical consequences express the impersonal reality of the social order. They also result in the power of individuals to make choices.

- Punishment is rarely tied in to the misbehavior. Logical consequences are logically related to misbehavior.

- Punishment tells children they are bad. Logical consequences imply no element of moral judgment.

- Punishment focuses on what is past. Logical consequences are concerned with present and future behavior.

- Punishment is associated with a threat, either open or concealed. Logical consequences are based on support and good will, not retaliation.

- Punishment is inconsistent, depending on the whim of the parent. Logical consequences are consistent because they arise from laws of nature and society.

- Punishment demands submission. Logical consequences permit choice.

Applying natural consequences

When parents begin to apply natural, logical consequences, they need to think through, in advance, how they are going to present the consequences and how they are going to follow through. Steps in applying natural consequences are:

- Choose meaningful natural consequences that impact children directly.

- Choose logical consequences that have minimal impact on parents.

- Explain meaningful consequences for children's behaviors in advance so they select from these consequences.

- Present consequences with kindness.

- Present choices with firmness.

- Follow through as planned. If you are not consistent, you undermine the system and teach children it is okay to not be responsible.

- Accept children's decisions with the choices they make. Remember, they had a choice. Parents need to detach and let go.

- Assure children that they may try again for the more positive consequences they desire. Make clear, however, how they will logically earn them by different behaviors.

- Be patient. It will take time for natural and logical consequences to be effective.

Presenting meaningful choices

We all make choices every day based on meaningful consequences. We are motivated for more difficult or unpleasant tasks if we associate them with pleasant consequences. For example, there may be parts of our job that we do not like, but we are motivated by the paycheck that lets us pay the mortgage, eat, and have some fun. We may also enjoy internal rewards from a job such as feeling responsible, helping others, and contributing on a team. Our job may also be helping us develop certain skills we want to improve. All of these motivate us to be responsible in our jobs. These rewards are meaningful to us.

Children also need meaningful consequences to help them be responsible. In fact, this is even more important for children because they are, by definition, immature. They need to learn how to be responsible in order to be mature. They are not as good at delaying gratification or working for internal satisfaction as adults. They ask, "Why should I do this?" because whatever the task, it does not seem to be meaningful.

When parents are helping children be responsible by giving them meaningful choices, it is important to look at what would motivate them. Some children, especially alcoholics/addicts, tend to be motivated more by external consequences such as not going to jail, losing a job, or having to move out of the house. Those who are not addicts/alcoholics may also be motivated by external consequences. They are more motivated for unpleasant tasks such as homework or cleaning their rooms when they get better grades, earn time with a parent to play a game, go for ice cream, earn points toward free time, or time to play their music.

Parents can help their children be motivated by more internal rewards, such as feeling good because you are helping a team, helping improve mankind, or being responsible. This will occur if parents praise their children for their positive, responsible behaviors. Many parents do not give enough praise, however, and they wonder why their children are not internally motivated. A mother describes how she learned the importance of praising her daughter:

When we brought our daughter into treatment, one of the first things that I heard in our parent group is that kids need a lot of praise. Our parent-group counselor said that the ratio should be 10 to 1, positive to negative. She said that praise would be a way to help kids feel good about what they were doing and develop an internal sense of pleasure for their hard work. It would also help them to be more responsible.

I thought I praised my kids, but when I really looked at this I saw that I took a lot of their positive behavior for granted. I focused on the negative. In fact, they got a lot of attention for their negative behavior. I learned that negative attention motivated them to act out, because at least I noticed them.

I had to look at how to give them attention for positives. I also needed to learn to say things like, "You are being responsible, and that's great," or "You are really helping us, and we appreciate it."

Contracts and natural consequences

Contracts are useful as a general parenting technique as well as in helping children with a self-corrective device when they have misbehaved. When families have written contracts where rules and consequences are spelled out, it is easier for children to know what is expected and what they are choosing. They know, for example, that they can choose between being in on time and earning points for music, or being late and losing these points as well as a percentage of their allowance. They know what is positive behavior, and they know what to choose as an alternative to negative behavior.

Contracts can be written to include such things as the use of drugs and alcohol, chores, borrowing of clothes, TV time, telephone time, curfew, respectful language, neatness in the home, respectful and non-violent behavior, smoking, and time with the family. On the latter, for example, it could be written on the contract that there is to be family time for three hours on a weekend afternoon. Someone in the family plans an outing each week. If anyone misses this event, the consequence could be that they serve breakfast in bed to each family member for three mornings the next week in addition to planning the next outing.

In this case, as in others, the negative consequences should be as close to the behavior as possible. Children and adolescents can then learn that consequences are logical.

All members of the family should be involved in setting up the contract. Children of all ages have creative ideas about meaningful consequences that parents may not think of, because children, or their siblings, know what is meaningful to them. The contract should also include everyone in the family; parents do chores and they also have consequences if they have violent, disrespectful behavior. This helps children learn that consequences are fair and for the benefit of the whole family.

Natural consequences and the addict

As discussed in Chapter 1, *Use, Abuse, and Dependency*, and Chapter 2, *Patterns of Development*, addicts/alcoholics will do whatever they can to continue the lifestyle that supports their love relationship with mood-altering substances. They will have denial, delusion, and rationalization about how their use affects them and others. The only thing that can motivate them to change is for them to believe that their drug/alcohol use has negative consequences they want to avoid. They perpetuate their drug-using lifestyle by denying the reality of their consequences. They are out of practice in facing reality. They live with the delusion that they will get their way if they lie and manipulate. Parents will have to work very hard on not making this a reality.

Parents who are not knowledgeable about addiction/alcoholism and working their own recovery programs will usually have more difficulty applying natural consequences. Chapter 6, *Harmful Consequences from Normal Feelings*, describes how codependency causes parents to fall into parenting traps and enable. Undoing this is a long process, but it is possible if parents work on it. A mother describes how she learned about logical natural consequences and how she and her husband applied them:

> At the beginning, we didn't know that our daughter was using, but when her behaviors started to fall apart we implemented new rules. We said that we would take the car away or ground her, but we hadn't always followed through before, so she did whatever she wanted. She totally disregarded any threats of consequences.
>
> We began to suspect that she was using, but I let myself get trapped in thinking that if I were a better mother, she wouldn't disobey me. She had all these zingers that I was the fault of her problems, and I just took them on. I was also ashamed of what was going on, so I wanted to keep it a secret. This meant that I didn't want to talk about it with outsiders.

Even though I had heard about Families Anonymous and Al-Anon, I didn't want to let my secrets out by even showing up at those meetings.

My husband and I started to fight a lot about what to do with our daughter. I was an emotional wreck, and I decided to see a therapist. As time went on, and her behaviors at home were getting worse, I started going to Families Anonymous at the suggestion of my therapist. That's when I started to learn what had worked for other parents. For example, I learned that we needed outside leverage since my daughter was disregarding home rules.

We went to her school and told them that we were on the same page with the consequences they had there like suspensions and detentions. We also said that we would be upset if they looked the other way when our daughter deserved these consequences.

Then we got involved with the lower level magistrate court system when our daughter was caught trespassing. This is relatively new in our community, and it was great to have the court involved at this level.

It wasn't long before she was charged with possession of drugs and drug paraphernalia, and possession of stolen goods. We worked closely with the courts, and that was a big relief. We had the leverage we needed. The natural consequence for her was that she had a court-ordered assessment and court-ordered treatment.

She tried to manipulate us in treatment to bring in things that were not allowed like candy and cigarettes and letters from drug-using friends, but we told her in advance that we knew the rules and we weren't going to help her break them. She tested us so many times until she learned that she was responsible for her behavior. We had to keep reminding her of the rules and her consequences.

Learning about consequences was a breakthrough for me. Now I know how to use outside consequences, but I have also learned about how to apply them in my own home. You have to be able to follow through, however. This is where the work on you starts. When you work on how you get codependent and fall in those parenting traps, you start to get better. All of this is so much easier when you have done the work on your own recovery.

Parents often struggle with how to select meaningful consequences. A father describes what he and his wife did, and how their school and court system helped:

In the beginning, the hardest thing we had to deal with as parents was how to come up with consequences that didn't affect the parents. The ones we used when [the teenagers] were younger, such as grounding, were harder on us than just letting them go out. We had to stay in the house, and we seemed to get in shouting matches with them when they yelled from their rooms that they wanted to be set free.

We learned to avoid the power struggles by having the kids face their consequences in the court system. This meant that we let them know in advance that we would file unruly and runaway and theft charges if their behaviors continued. It was their choice. The court system worked the best for us because the court system applied the consequences, and they directly affected the children.

There were still some ways that we were affected, but they were less than getting into power struggles with the kids. For example, the courts made them wear ankle bracelets to monitor their whereabouts. A machine was wired from the courthouse to check in every twenty minutes. This tied the phone up. It made it hard for us to have our own extended conversations.

We also learned to use natural consequences and let our children be responsible for their relationship with the courts and the police and even their school.

The children knew that we wouldn't be there to negotiate for them or to get them off. We also were not going to listen to their complaints about the school or the teachers.

We were fortunate to have a school system and a court system that cared enough about kids to not enable them. Parents sometimes have to help this along by saying they believe in consequences as a way to help kids. So many parents try to get their kids off. Schools these days get scared that parents will complain if they follow through with applying the rules that the kids know they have broken. Schools need our support. The partnership really worked for us.

When teenagers drop out of school, however, this type of leverage is not available. A mother shares how she and her husband applied natural consequences to help their substance-abusing son when he dropped out:

We didn't use school leverage like we could have, and we made some mistakes because we didn't know better. The end result was that we had no leverage to move our son into treatment until things got even worse.

He finally dropped out of school, just like he was dropping out of everything else, including respect for his parents. He was in charge of the house, and it was like we were prisoners. Consequences and rules made no difference to him.

Then he had problems with the police. We had started going to meetings at Families Anonymous, and we were much stronger and more knowledgeable about what to do. Our son couldn't manipulate us as easily.

We started to give our son choices and apply natural consequences when he was about to have his first court hearing. We told him that he had a choice to go to the hearing, and if he did not it would make his eventual court consequences even worse.

We also told him that if he did choose to go, he had to arrange his own transportation. We were not going to leave work even earlier to come home to pick him up for a 3:00 hearing. It was more a consequence for us to lose even more time from work. We decided that it was really his court hearing, his consequence.

We presented him with the choice that he could either take the bus from home, or he could drive with one of us to work at 7 a.m. and wait in a coffee shop all day until we drove to the hearing. We also made sure that we had something else to do after the hearing, so he had to find a way home for himself. We said this to him with kindness and respect, and not with a lecture.

The next way we applied natural, logical consequences was to give him choices about living at home. He was almost 18, so this made it easier for us to have him move out, but parents can often emancipate their children if they are younger.

We gave him the choice of living at home with three basic rules: no drugs, no obscene pornography lying around, and no violence. He was using, of course, so he couldn't obey those rules. The consequence was that he had to leave or go to treatment. He chose to leave.

His big natural consequence was that he had to get a job with enough money to pay the rent, and he had to do his clothes at a laundromat, stuff like that. He tried to get us to rescue him a few times, and we had to be careful not to do it. He wanted the creature comforts at home, but he wasn't willing to be in recovery to help himself to earn them. He was still in a me, me, and me stage.

The amazing thing is that over time he has gotten better at personal responsibility, and he even says that he isn't using because it interferes with his goals. He never had any goals before, so we see that he has learned by his own consequences that what he does with his life, good or bad, is up to him. He seemed to have a sense of what the behaviors were that were getting him into trouble. If we had rescued him, he never would have learned this.

When parents improve their knowledge and understanding of addiction and alcoholism, it is easier to see how they are helping their addict/alcoholic by encouraging them to face the reality of their choices. A father talks about this issue:

One of the consequences of our son's drug and alcohol abuse was that we could not trust him with our car. We also knew that earning driving privileges would be one of the most meaningful consequences for positive behavior.

We set up some simple rules that would allow him to drive, such as he needed to have a C average at school and he had to have a job so that he could pay his portion of the car insurance.

His drug and alcohol use was more important to him, however, so he never earned driving privileges. We couldn't understand the power of addiction before Families Anonymous, but we came to understand the choice he was making. We had to accept what the disease was in order to let go. That gave us a lot of freedom to apply other natural consequences.

Our son was a sick person, not a bad person. He needed to see that his sickness was using drugs and that he had negative consequences from this. He eventually saw that he wanted to change, and he is in the process of doing this today. He still hasn't earned driving privileges, but he is moving closer to that goal. We are there to support him in whatever positive choices he makes.

I used to look at newspaper articles about kids in trouble and wonder how parents could ever let this happen. Now that it has happened to me, I see how the kids get themselves into trouble. Parents need to move out of their shame and help their children look at the reality of their lives.

When addicts/alcoholics start to get better, it is important that parents continue to use natural consequences and not let their teenagers have privileges before they earn them. A mother relates how trust can be earned:

Our daughter had really improved with recovery from the old days when she was so out of control, but she wanted all of her privileges at once. For example, she wanted unlimited use of the car, and she was real boo-hoo about it when we said no. She had been able to push the "feel sorry for me" button in the past, but now her father and I were stronger. We told her that we cared about her, and we empathized with her frustration. But we were also firm that we needed to trust that she could be responsible with the car. We said that she could use it to go to and from AA meetings and then, if she were responsible with that for six weeks, she would earn more time. This seemed to work, and she did earn more time.

When parents are not strong in their own recoveries, it is easy to return to old parenting traps and enabling. A father describes how easy it is to slip and what can happen:

We learned how to make a home contract when our son was in a month of residential treatment, and we started to implement it as soon as he came home. He was now in outpatient at the same agency. After about a week of positive behaviors, he told us that he didn't need the contract anymore. He also said that despite what his outpatient counselor said, he didn't need the kind of structure that everyone was giving him. He said that we were right back to controlling him, and working his recovery for him, and we were not using what we had learned in Families Anonymous.

We were not very strong, so we believed him. We started to let things slip on the contract. We didn't tell the staff at the outpatient program because we were confused. We also were embarrassed that our son wasn't as welcoming of structure as some of the other kids in his treatment group. We were afraid that if the treatment program knew what was happening, they would kick him out.

We soon found out that our son had relapsed shortly after leaving residential treatment. This is why he started the old addict's blame game where everything he did was right and everything we did was wrong. When addicts want privileges so soon after they enter recovery, it is a good sign that they are not working a recovery program and they even may have relapsed. Parents need to be aware of this.

It was also amazing to me how easily my wife and I got back to the old parenting traps and enabling behaviors. Our parent-group counselor had said that she didn't cure us, just like we can't cure the addict. I had sort of thought that she did cure me, however. I learned that I was going to have to do a lot of work on my codependency.

Sometimes parents have to apply what they have learned about natural consequence to older brothers or sisters who are away at college when a family enters recovery back home. These older siblings may be abusing drugs and alcohol and need a strong message about their own consequences. A mother explains how she and her husband intervened with a college-age brother:

We came to treatment with our addict/alcoholic daughter in high school, but we began to appreciate that we needed to present her brother in college with some new choices. We knew that he was abusing alcohol and drugs because he had done this with his younger sister. We also knew that since he was away from home, we had a different kind of challenge.

We told him that if our financial support was going to continue, he had to have a C average and not have legal charges. We also told him that when he came home, he could not use drugs or alcohol in the house, and he could not engage in either verbal or physical intimidation. He was also told not to destroy the property in and around the house and that he was responsible to keep his own room neat and clean.

He was told all of this in a written contract with the consequence of staying in school and living at home on vacations clearly laid out if he chose them by positive behaviors. It was also stated that if he violated any of the home expectations, he was expected to be out in four days.

The interesting thing is that he chose not to live at home as soon as we presented the contract. He has maintained his grades, but we will see how long that lasts. He knows we will follow through, and that his behaviors have consequences. We see this as helping him learn responsibility.

Parents also see that having structure and consequences is necessary to maintain quality in their own lives, apart from how this structure might be helping their impulse-driven, drug/alcohol-abusing, and dependent teenagers. A father describes what can happen when parents stop giving their children of all ages everything they want:

> It is important for parents to be saying to their kids that this is how they want to be living their lives. There are ways they want to sleep, for example, and these don't include kids having parties or coming in at late hours and being disruptive. Kids need to hear that their parents have needs, and that their lives don't totally revolve around what their kids want.

> Kids don't always like to hear this, but part of their immaturity is that they think the whole world revolves around what they want. Kids notice a change in us when we are less codependent, and they may rebel. But we are working on ourselves, what we can change. This is pretty exciting.

Gifts from natural consequences

Families start to change when there is a clear understanding of natural consequences. Also, long-term recovery means that parents and addicts/alcoholics realize the consequences of their hard work.

Changes for families

Family members find it easier to live with each other when they act more respectfully in the house. It is easier to function without using defenses when there are natural and logical consequences for negative behaviors.

Chapter 7, *Communication and Relationships*, discusses the chaos that occurs when family roles are taken on to deal with the stress of practicing alcoholics/addicts. Family heroes overcompensate for this chaos, as do the prosecutors, the super parents, the lost children, and the rebellious children. Alcoholics/addicts rule the household and codependent parents are not strong enough to stop them.

When parents become strong enough to apply consequences for out-of-control behavior and do not allow themselves to be manipulated by their teenage substance abusers, this may also improve their relationship with their other children. A mother discusses how her family changed their patterns of relating:

> As my husband and I got stronger, we began to see that we owed it to our two daughters to not enable their addict/alcoholic brother any longer. The family had gotten into some very unhealthy patterns as a result of adapting to his drug abuse. This realization helped us to follow through with what we needed to do to help the whole family.

> We learned in treatment about how the roles were a result of the stress we had in the family. Now it was up to us to do things differently and to take a new kind of leadership in our family. We were determined to not go back to the old days, so we used everything we had learned to move forward.

Changes for parents

When parents first learn about the importance of natural consequences for addicts/alcoholics, they focus on how to apply them with their substance-abusing teenagers and their other children. As their skills progress, they see how applying consequences is even more far reaching and significant in their overall personal growth. The mother of an addict tells how she changed with her ex-husband and her friends:

> When I started to work on letting go of my fixing behaviors, I realized that I needed to make clear to people that there would be consequences for things they did that they would have to take care of, not me. This started with my recovering daughter, of course, in terms of any trouble she would get in. But then I started to apply what I had learned with my ex-husband and my friends.

> I had been so good at bailing people out of their consequences that I had to work extra hard on this. In the first place, I had to work hard on taking responsibility for myself. I had to stop the fact that I let myself get pulled in by other people who wanted me to fix their problems. I had to pay attention to my triggers such as the need to be liked no matter what. I was the one inviting people to ask for things, and I really couldn't blame them.

> Then I had to make it clear to my friends that I wasn't going to pay their rent if they spent their money. I wasn't going to baby-sit their kids if

they forgot about appointments and didn't get a sitter. I wasn't going to drive their big dog to the kennel because they hadn't planned enough time for this before leaving on vacation. These are examples of things I had done. People needed to plan ahead and experience their own consequences. Their crisis didn't need to be mine.

I also told my ex-husband that if he didn't show up for a preplanned visit with our son, he was going to have to take care of explaining it. I was going to take myself out of the middle. I learned to say to my son that he needed to tell his dad how it affected him, and that I wasn't going to speak for him. It was a consequence for his father, and his father needed to face it. I figured that it was also good for my son to learn how to tell others how their behavior made him feel. This is a good life skill.

I found that people were a bit confused with this at the beginning because I had been so good at the rescue routine, but I kept going and they got the message. It was amazing to me that they started to get better organized and more responsible themselves. I realized that I hadn't really been helping them as much as I thought except that I was helping to cripple them.

Parents in recovery learn to not react like they used to. A mother explains how not reacting has helped her:

The more I looked at natural consequences and how they work, I realized that I didn't have to automatically stop in my tracks and take on the consequences of others' feelings and behaviors in terms of words that they would dish out to me. I hadn't realized that if people said things, I didn't need to take them on.

For example, I didn't need to take on the comments that other people were making about me. Those words were theirs and didn't need to be mine. I could say, "Thank you for sharing," but then I could stop and say to myself, "check list," to review what they said and ask myself if it fit. I didn't need to take on their words automatically.

I have to be careful that I don't dismiss feedback prematurely, of course, but I have also realized that just because someone says something, I don't have to own it. I look at what garbage is mine and what is theirs. For example, one friend was really good at dishing out stuff with her anger because she had had a bad day or something. One time she

called me in one of her moods and said that she was coming over. I told
her not to, but I knew she would anyway since I had let her dump on me
in the past. This time I wrote a note and put it on the front door that said,
"I am taking no more deliveries at this time." I watched her read it from
the upstairs window, and she tore it up. She was learning, though, and I
had to take responsibility for teaching her that her frustration was her
consequence. I wasn't willing to accept the consequence of her taking out
her feelings on me.

Sometimes people want to give you their garbage. You don't have to
take it. I have healthier boundaries now.

In Al-Anon I learned that I don't have to react immediately to what
people say or do. I can slow down and look at what happened, or what
they said. I can also remove myself from situations ahead of time when I
anticipate consequences that I do not choose to take.

This consequences stuff was so freeing for me. It started with work-
ing on applying natural consequences to help my addict son in recovery,
but it went on to help me with all the relationships in my life. I never
would have thought this when I started. It went way beyond what I was
doing with my addict son.

Changes for addicts/alcoholics

Adolescent alcoholics/addicts in recovery know they need structure and
accountability to continue to improve themselves. They know the power of
their disease. They also know that holding on to meaningful goals helps
them move forward.

In Chapter 8, *Working on Recovery*, recovering alcoholics/addicts describe
how having a tough sponsor and having the court and their treatment program on their backs helps them. Addicts with more than fifteen years of
sobriety tell their stories in that chapter. Another teen who went through
treatment relates how she has come a long way thanks to positive choices
and outsiders holding her accountable:

I had a lot to work on in residential treatment twenty years ago. I
was an addict/alcoholic, but I also had a psychiatric illness so I had a
dual-diagnosis.

One of the first things that happened in treatment was that someone on the staff I respected sat me down when I was acting out in my psychiatric stuff. She said that I had the choice of being in a mental ward all my life or living a normal life where I had a job and an apartment like other people. She was really tough with me, but she had tears in her eyes when she told me because she cared so much. It was twenty years ago, but I still remember where we were sitting and how the birds sounded. She was the director of this program, and it even made more of an impact that she sought me out because I knew that she was busy.

It also made an impact because she said that she believed in me, and I could choose health if I really wanted it. It was up to me. It was easier for me to be sick and to feel sorry for myself, but I wanted those consequences of an apartment and a job where I could live a responsible life and be on my own.

I kept going, and what really helped is that a judge was on my back as well as my parents. I was not being enabled, so every time I tried to manipulate, it didn't work. It was tempting to slip back, but it was almost impossible because I knew that I would have negative consequences.

I am in my early 30s now, and I have a good job and my own apartment. I went back to my treatment program last year for a reunion and saw the woman who sat me down twenty years ago. I said that I hadn't forgotten our talk. What surprised me is that she said she hadn't forgotten it either. She even had the same tears in her eyes when she told me.

Taking care of yourself

This chapter illustrates that if parents work on not enabling their children and their substance-abusing teenagers, they will help themselves as well as their entire family. The chapter also shares stories of parents who formed a partnership with the schools and the courts in order to maximize the help they could give to their substance abusers. Parents are encouraged to use this knowledge to make their own partnerships. A mother who spoke earlier gives her encouragement:

After one of our court hearings, I told my daughter's probation officer that I supported the consequences from the courts. He, like the principal, complimented me.

I realized, again, that there are a lot of enabling parents out there who are making it more difficult for schools and even courts to help kids face their consequences and bottom out so they start to get well. No wonder courts and schools get scared to follow up. We need to reach out and say that we support them and we need their help. They need to hear from us that we do not want them to enable our kids.

CHAPTER 11

Stories of Empowerment

The rewards for those who persevere far
exceed the pain that must precede the victory.

—Ted Engstrom

WHEN PARENTS ARE STRUGGLING because they suspect that their teenagers are abusing alcohol and drugs, they can feel angry, confused, burnt out, and hopeless. Police cars may be coming to their home, and school truancy officers or principals may be calling them at work. In addition, they may feel like prisoners in their own homes, afraid to come out.

Once parents learn more about drug/alcohol abuse and dependency, how to get an assessment, how to choose an appropriate treatment program, how to work on their own feelings and the destructive communication patterns that have become habits in their homes, and how to reach out for help in recovery, they begin to find a new freedom and a new happiness.

This new way of life is possible for all parents of drug/alcohol abusers or addicts/alcoholics, whether or not their adolescents are sober, drug free, and in recovery. Those parents who choose the challenge of developing recovery programs are promised rewards they never thought possible. The mother of an adolescent addict explains:

> *My husband and I are enjoying our lives without being wrapped in that tight cocoon of substance abuse and dependency where the whole family can't move or breathe. We believed in the promises of recovery from the very beginning, and they have kept us going. Our lives changed dramatically when we started to work on codependency and added the structure of the Twelve Steps, the slogans, and the Serenity Prayer.*

The stories in this chapter will show how people in recovery chose to empower themselves.

Living the Twelve Steps

As described in Chapter 8, *Working on Recovery*, the Twelve Steps are the organizing principles of recovery for adolescents and their parents. As parents grow in recovery, they talk about going beyond *working* on the steps to actually *living* them. Each Step is a guide to daily behavior that will improve serenity and lead toward empowerment.

Since the stories in this chapter often reference a particular Step by number, we will list the Twelve Steps here (rather than sending you to other chapters):

The Twelve Steps[1]

1. *We admitted we were powerless over alcohol—that our lives had become unmanageable.*

2. *Came to believe that a Power greater than ourselves could restore us to sanity.*

3. *Made a decision to turn our will and our lives over to the care of God, as we understood Him.*

4. *Made a searching and fearless moral inventory of ourselves.*

5. *Admitted to God, to ourselves and to another human being, the exact nature of our wrongs.*

6. *Were entirely ready to have God remove all these defects of character.*

7. *Humbly asked Him to remove our shortcomings.*

8. *Made a list of all persons we had harmed and became willing to make amends to them all.*

9. *Made direct amends to such people wherever possible, except when to do so would injure them or others.*

10. *Continued to take personal inventory and when we were wrong, promptly admitted it.*

11. *Sought through prayer and meditation to improve our conscious contact with God, as we understood Him, praying only for knowledge of His will for us and the power to carry that out.*

12. *Having had a spiritual awakening as a result of these Steps, we tried to carry this message to others and to practice these principles in all our affairs.*

As parents develop stronger and stronger recoveries, they are able to live the Steps in their daily lives. Living the Steps does not mean that the parents are perfect, however. The program of recovery believes in progress, not perfection. These stories illustrate how this works as several parents comment on their experience with Steps One and Ten:

> As my daughter has moved through her 20s and now into her early 30s, I have to come back to the First Step when I start to remind her about going to AA meetings or working her program. I do this out of fear because she has such a good life. I get scared that she is going to throw it all away. I have to remember all the things I have heard about living the Twelve Steps and hold my tongue. This is a lot easier for me now because I have worked on accepting that I did not cause, I cannot control, and I cannot cure her, but part of living this Step is accepting it every day.

· · · · ·

> I have been going to Al-Anon meetings for a number of years since our addicted child went to treatment, and it is amazing to me how much I have to continue to pay attention to the First Step. Some days I am really strong, but on others I slip and my old controlling comes back. In living my program, I challenge myself to be humble and to admit that I need to revisit all of the Steps. I do so, and I really appreciate the structure they offer me. It's like I need to look at the map again and retrace my path. Then I get back on the road that I want to be on.

· · · · ·

> Step Ten has been such a great help to me in giving me the structure to not return to my old ways. I like to think of the choices I have, and this empowers me to be excited about choosing to say that I was wrong, that I let my fears get in the way of letting go, or that I didn't follow through with something like I wanted to.

> I have also worked on not judging myself if I am not perfect, and this helps me to live this Step in my life. I put so much pressure on myself in the old days; to see myself as successful, I had to come up with the correct solution. If anything wasn't going right in my life or anyone else's, it was my job to fix it. I even deluded myself to think that I always had the right answers. Boy, was that ever a set-up! I was not a humble person.

> Living the Tenth Step is a great way to avoid a return to that pressure and loneliness I created for myself because no one wanted to be

around the arrogant person I became. People have told me that I am so much more approachable today. I even get compliments on my humility. This shows me what happens when I live the Tenth Step.

As parents grow in their recovery, the last section of the Twelfth Step is often the most challenging and relevant in terms of what it means to live the Steps as part of a recovery program. The father of an addict explains how this section has inspired him:

> *The statement in the Twelfth Step about practicing these principles in all our affairs really inspires me after seventeen years in recovery. It has probably stayed with me more than anything else in the program of recovery. Just as I believe that the alcoholic will not change unless they change their lifestyle, the same is true for codependents, us family members in recovery. We must practice the Steps in all our affairs.*
>
> *What I have worked on is choosing happiness, not being judgmental, and not trying to control other people. I have had to really surrender to this and work hard on it.*
>
> *Part of living the Steps is to not just let myself give lip service to them. I have to be tough on myself and hold myself accountable. I like this because then I can earn respect for myself. I want to be able to say that I practice what I preach.*

Practicing the Serenity Prayer

Many parents of addicts/alcoholics find that daily use of the Serenity Prayer helps them to live recovery. They work hard on practicing the prayer, especially during the most difficult times.

Several parents tell stories of how they have used this prayer to live their recovery:

> *When our daughter went to treatment several years ago, we said the Serenity Prayer at the end of our therapy groups. I didn't relate to not being able to change things at first because I am one of those action-oriented people. I never give up. I am sort of like a dog that won't let go of the bone. This trait has helped me a lot in my career. People know that they can count on me to not give up early. The Serenity Prayer seemed to be for wimps.*

I was resistant to everything about recovery because I thought that alcoholism and addiction were my daughter's problems, not mine. I had a very successful career, and I didn't really have anything about myself to work on. I went to Al-Anon because I didn't want anyone at our treatment program to think that I wasn't a good parent, but I sat in the meetings and planned my work week or thought about a difficult conference call I had had that day.

As time went on, I respected some of the people I met in Al-Anon because they had accomplished a lot in their lives. They were high-energy people like me. One of them told their story in a meeting about what the Serenity Prayer meant in their life, and I was amazed. I had never thought about how a high-powered executive could use it.

I look back on this and have to laugh because I was so arrogant about what I thought I knew. I was also so judgmental. My life changed when I heard someone in my own fast lane tell their story, but then I started to learn how to get the same strength and hope from others who were not like me.

I had to work on accepting what I cannot change in a spiritual way that respects others for who they are without judging them. I see now that changing what I can means that I still have goals. But I also need to focus on aspects of myself that I need to change.

I need to focus on my arrogance all the time. I can still slip back into judgments. Now I catch myself more often before I make a sarcastic remark. I say the Serenity Prayer backwards to give me time to hold my tongue. I am a lot happier today than I was when my daughter started treatment. It has really helped to practice the Serenity Prayer in my daily life.

· · · · ·

When I first came in recovery, I used a lot of what I was learning to help me with my alcoholic teenager. Even though the focus was on me, it was about how to practice the prayer in relation to alcoholism. The thing I could not change was my son's alcoholism. I could only change myself.

As my recovery deepened, I was using the Serenity Prayer in other aspects of my life. The Twelfth Step talks about putting all the Steps into practice in all of your everyday affairs, and I tried to do this with the

Serenity Prayer as well. If I was really going to practice the prayer, I needed to do it with all the members of my family and with my colleagues at work, with friends, neighbors, and even with God when I would question God's will in my life. It was the goal of my recovery to have more serenity in my life. In order to achieve this goal, I had to continually sort out what I could not change and those things that I could.

Again and again, I would come back to the fact that what I could change is myself and what I could not change is other people. I have worked on accepting how other people behave, but I have worked on having the courage to change my own behavior. I have come to know more and more serenity as I have worked on this. It is a lifelong journey, but I get excited about how even better I will be a year from now.

Living the slogans

Those outside of recovery will often see slogans like *One Day at a Time* on the bumper ahead of them at a traffic light. These slogans, and a handful of others, are used as reminders in recovery of some profound principles. Parents who have empowered themselves show how they live these slogans in their daily lives.

"Easy Does It"

Two parents describe how they use the slogan "Easy Does It" to remind themselves to back off and relax:

When I started recovery several years ago, I felt like I was fighting in a war. Each battle was so difficult, yet I did not want to be defeated. I thought I was fighting a battle against drugs and alcohol and all the bad things associated with addiction, but I realized that I was fighting a war against myself. I was getting nowhere. The war was in all my control tactics. I finally started to give up the fight and practice "Easy Does It."

· · · · ·

The slogan that has meant the most to me is "Easy Does It."

It was so easy for me to be a perfectionist and get so wrapped up with things and overdo. It would drive my family crazy. My kids and my husband would even say that I didn't need to prepare that grand of a dinner or clean the house like we had a ten-person cleaning service.

Today I know that a lot of that frantic activity was a way to escape my fears about my son's addiction. When I started to work on understanding the disease and facing my fears, I didn't have to put so much energy into denying them.

Part of living recovery for me is being so much more relaxed. I make decisions every day that certain things are not important to me, whereas in the old days everything was important. People say that I am a much nicer person to be around.

"One Day at a Time"

Several parents describe how they use the slogan "One Day at a Time" to help them break tasks down and live in the present:

When my teenager went into treatment, and I first heard the slogans, I thought they were so trite. I had seen them as bumper stickers, and I thought they were so simplistic.

As time went on and I was trying to work a recovery program, however, I loved the slogans. "One Day at a Time" meant a lot to me, especially when things seem so enormous. In the beginning of recovery, I applied this to the challenge of not controlling my alcoholic teenager and letting go that I could not cure addiction and make it go away. I knew this was true. I decided that I could believe it one day at a time. Each morning I would pray that I could practice this idea for that particular day.

Later, I lived the slogan in a number of ways. One in particular was when I decided to return to a goal that I had before we had addiction in our family, and go to graduate school. This was a bit overwhelming to me because I had to write a thesis. I broke it down into small parts, however, and focused on completing one part in a day without dwelling on my fears of what lay ahead. It helped me tremendously, and I am proud to say that I competed the thesis and got my graduate degree with honors.

The slogan "One Day at a Time" has helped me with lots of challenges. It is a way I live my life.

• • • • •

I really use the slogan "One Day at a Time" in my recovery program.

First of all, I try to live my life in day-tight compartments and not focus on the past or the future. This was helpful at the beginning when I worried a lot about our addict teenager or when I thought about all the misery that she caused in the past. I was not free to pay attention to what she was doing in the here and now.

By focusing on one day, I could notice the good things and I was also more alert to what her old manipulations were that used to lead to my enabling her. I could make better choices in the here and now with freedom from the past and future worries. My decisions were better.

The next thing I focused on was recognizing the gifts in every day. I had stopped paying attention to things like flowers, sunsets, or laughter. I had stopped looking people in the eye. I had stopped taking time to smile at the children I passed on a playground. I started to celebrate these things.

After all, every day is a gift. That's why it is called the present.

"How Important Is It?"

Two parents describe how the slogan "How Important Is It?" helps them keep a healthy perspective on what is important in their lives:

"How Important Is It?" has been my favorite slogan over years of trying to live my recovery since our then-teenager went to addiction treatment.

When I was growing up in an alcoholic family, worry was the way we operated. Worry was passed down to me as if it was necessary. You couldn't live without it.

Recovery has changed everything for me. When I start worrying, and start controlling over the smallest of things, I think of the slogan and ask the question of how important something is in the grand scheme of things. This helps me to detach and let go. It helps me a lot with control.

• • • • •

I really like the slogan "How Important Is It?" because it helps me remember that I have had a lot of worries in my life, but most of them have never happened.

Before I started to really live a recovery program, I would ruin my day by worrying about the future. Oftentimes, the things I worried about never happened. I have to focus on staying in the present and thinking about how important that is. I say to myself that it isn't important to worry about something in the future that may never happen.

"Live and Let Live"

A mother describes how she uses the slogan "Live and Let Live" to maintain healthier relationships:

> The most important slogan for me since I began recovery about seventeen years ago is "Live and Let Live." This was initially tied into all the work I was doing on my spiritual program and what I needed to let go of since I lived with a lot of fear that our teenager would not be sober and drug-free. I kept going on my personal work, however, because I knew that it wasn't about what our child would do, it was about what I needed to work on for myself.
>
> Our child did enter recovery for many years. When he relapsed, entered recovery, and relapsed again, I got back into some of my old controlling and the old roller coaster rides. My program was really being tested.
>
> It has been important for me to accept who my child is, and to respect the fight that an addict has with addiction. The addict's consequences are theirs to deal with, not mine.
>
> I have to focus on not calling my child to ask about going to meetings, or to get details on how his time is being spent. I did that for a while and found that he was not only abrupt, and wanted to end our conversation, but our relationship was so strained that it almost ended.
>
> My child is working on getting stronger, but that is something I have let go of. He calls me now, asks me about my life, and it is wonderful. I love him, and I know that he loves me. He seems to appreciate that I respect him enough to let go. I just try to focus on letting him live his own life.

"Let Go and Let God"

Four parents describe how the slogan "Let Go and Let God" has helped them find acceptance, peace, and strength in their lives:

The slogan that has meant the most to me ever since the early days when I started going to Al-Anon is "Let Go and Let God." I was in so much pain in the early days over what was going on, and the idea that I could let go of that pain and that God would take it, meant so much to me. I could also let go of all the craziness that alcoholism brings.

• • • • •

I have been able to live recovery by using the slogan "Let Go and Let God." It is easy to remember, and when I think about it I am reminded of the Twelve Steps. It ties into how I have worked on the Steps, and the journey I have been on.

At the beginning, the slogan helped me to let go of what my addicted teenager was doing by not engaging in fights with him because I had so much rage. I would stand upstairs and pray for strength to go downstairs and not make matters worse by yelling. I would ask God to take my anger, to help me calm down. This was possible because I had taken my inventory in the Fourth Step, worked on my anger, and saw that using it was a mistake for me, no matter how much I tried to justify it.

Later in recovery I have seen how letting go to God has helped in so many other ways such as letting go of my fears, letting go of what I think my limitations are in how far I can go in my career, and letting go of my judgments about other people. I turn these over to God. This helps me to grow and develop beyond what I could do on my own.

The meaning of "Let Go and Let God" has deepened over the years of recovery. I have tried to not use it as a cop-out where I just shrug my shoulders and toss off a slogan. That would not really be living the slogan; that isn't what it means. What it relates to are those times when you have done everything you can do, and you have worked hard, but you can't fix something, or solve something.

As the mother of grown children it is especially important for me to use the slogan. My children have their own lives. Sometimes I get scared, however. I know that they have challenges ahead. I picture them being held in God's hands with a bubble of light around them. God will take care of them, no matter what happens.

• • • • •

The slogan that has meant the most in living my recovery over many years is "Let Go and Let God" because I have had so much that I needed to let go in terms of alcoholism and addiction.

I had been struggling with controlling my husband's drinking for many years. I had become quite proficient in nagging, lecturing, screaming, threatening, crying, supervising, manipulating, insisting, giving in to, refusing to give in to, refusing to give up, and pretending that everything was perfect.

When my son began using alcohol and drugs, I used the same controlling techniques. I struggled in coming to terms with this. I didn't want to take my own inventory.

I kept using my old control, but nothing changed. Then I started letting go. I surrendered. It was hard at first because I thought I was giving up on my son and husband. It was as if I was a failure. I did not want to be a failure.

It did not mean I was a failure, however. It meant that I needed to work on myself. It did not mean I did not care about them or love them. It meant the opposite: I cared and loved them so much that this is what I needed to do. I did not have to tolerate their behavior. I had to set limits and boundaries.

My spouse continued to make choices that were not acceptable to me. Letting go of the marriage was healthy for me. It was a way to take care of myself, and to let him know that I was not willing to live in a sick relationship. He had his choice to continue his lifestyle, but I didn't need to do it with him.

I remember attending a Families Anonymous meeting when a mother was struggling with letting go. She said something like, "I guess I just love my daughter too much to let go. I can't do it; I am not a mean person." I told her that letting go is something that you do out of love. You let people or relationships go as a form of love and respect for what you cannot change. You turn them over to God.

· · · · ·

The slogan "Let Go and Let God" has meant so much to me in my life, and as my recovery deepens, it means even more. I have worked on turning over my impatience and judgments about others and myself and God has taken them. I heard a modified version of the Serenity Prayer at a Families Anonymous meeting that has really helped me. This is how it goes:

> God, grant me the serenity to accept the things I cannot change, the courage to change the things I can, and the wisdom to know the difference. Grant me patience with the things that take time, tolerance of the struggles of others that may be different from my own, appreciation for all that I have, and the willingness to get up and try again. I ask for this, one day at a time.

Believing in the promises of recovery

When the founders of AA wrote the *Big Book of Alcoholics Anonymous* in the late 1930s, they promised that the lives of suffering alcoholics would change if they followed a program of 12 step recovery. The founders were aware of skeptics, however, so they added a few words of encouragement:

> Are these extravagant promises? We think not. They are being fulfilled among us—sometimes quickly, sometimes slowly. They will always materialize if we work for them.[2]

The promises of recovery appear throughout the *Big Book*. Those written in the chapter called *Into Action* were previously noted in this book's Chapter 8. They are given again here so you can easily relate the stories that follow to the promises to which they are referring:[3]

> We are going to know a new freedom and a new happiness. We will not regret the past nor wish to shut the door on it. We will comprehend the word serenity and we will know peace. No matter how far down the scale we have gone, we will see how our experience can benefit others. That feeling of uselessness and self-pity will disappear. We will lose interest in selfish things and gain interest in our fellows. Self-seeking will slip away. Our whole attitude and outlook upon life will change. Fear of people and of economic insecurity will leave us. We will intuitively know how to handle situations which used to baffle us. We will suddenly realize that God is doing for us what we could not do for ourselves.

The following stories show how these promises are working in many lives. The first three stories are from an adolescent addict and his parents after one month of working a recovery program:

Before coming to my current treatment program, I was addicted to alcohol, marijuana, and opium, and I had many consequences. I had domestic violence and criminal damaging charges, and had been kicked out of a good Catholic school I was in. I was even kicked out of my first treatment program. I thought it was a joke, and I used alcohol and drugs all the time I was in it.

When I first came into treatment the second time, I was happy because I wasn't in jail, but I wasn't really thinking much beyond that. I wasn't really thinking about recovery or staying straight. I really didn't have any goals except having fun, and drugs were a way to have fun.

Now I am setting goals and planning on going to college. I was inspired by the promise in the Big Book *that my whole attitude and outlook on life would change if I followed abstinence and a program of recovery. I have a more positive attitude about life than I have ever had. I try to focus on clean, sober thinking, which is all about looking at the consequences of my choices for me and other people.*

My attitude in the past was "Leave me alone and let me do what I want." I was like, "I ain't doin' nuthin', and I don't care." I was really lying to myself because deep down I knew I was in trouble. I did care. I thought that I had to have this big bad boy image. Now I know that society doesn't look up to that. If you're going to make something of yourself, you can't think this way.

Now I'm trying to make something out of myself. Honesty is the best policy. One of the recovering staff says he lives his life with three basic principles: respect, care, and honesty. All those things will get you through. It's all about respecting others and caring about their situations. You need to face reality, and be honest with how it is in the world. I am trying to think about what I need to do if I am going to make something out of my life.

· · · · ·

The promise I relate to the most after one month of being in recovery is that we are going to know a new freedom and a new happiness. Since our son has been getting help, I have learned about the three Cs: that I didn't cause his drug use, that I can't cure it, and I can't control it. Each and every day I think about those when I start to go back to my old thinking, and I feel happy again.

· · · · ·

Even though I have been in recovery for only a month, I can already relate to the promise about how our whole attitude and outlook on life will change.

I should have had all my education about addiction 40 years ago and it would have saved me a lot of anger and heartache. Now I am learning what I cannot control, and how to let go and let God.

When we first brought our son into treatment a month ago, I was very upset that we were here. I didn't drink and I didn't do drugs and I had a lot of judgments about anyone who did, including my own son. I was also angry about having to come to family groups and a Saturday morning parent group because all of this was not my problem. I had grown up in an alcoholic home, and I had lived my life to make sure that I was not an alcoholic and addict. I felt that my son was letting me down because he couldn't stay away from drugs.

Then, in parent group, there was a lot of talk about what happens when you grow up in an alcoholic home like I did. The parent-group counselor even brought this little red chair to the group and asked us to imagine ourselves as a little kid sitting in it. She told us to imagine that we were looking up at the tall, out-of-control alcoholics in our lives. She got down on her knees with me to help me understand even more what being little was all about in my alcoholic home.

This was a real breakthrough for me. I started to think about the alcoholic parent I grew up with, and how my anger was covering up a lot of hurt. I also saw that my years of judging my parent, and judging my son, were from not understanding the disease.

If I had understood the disease earlier, I would have tried to help my son in different ways than I did. I had a hatred that made me stay away from my parent and, then, my son. Now I understand a lot more, and I am free of the hatred and the resentment. Now I am free to pray for them and not be judgmental. I am free to be compassionate. I am also free of all *the stress that my anger was causing. I am more relaxed with my son and my wife and my parents, and I am looking forward to my future.*

Parents who have been in family recovery for a while know that the promises of recovery can take on even deeper meaning as time passes. Parents who have been in recovery for at least two years now share their stories. Many of these parents have adolescents who have not chosen to be sober or drug-free, despite diagnoses of addiction and/or alcoholism:

The promise I relate to the most after two years in recovery is the one that says that your feelings of uselessness and self-pity will disappear.

When I first started my recovery, I had feelings of uselessness and depression. I despaired about how I must have done something wrong as a mother to have a drug addict for a child. Something must be terribly wrong with me. I had a lot of self-pity in this despair, too, because we had lived a good life and my husband and I were good parents. I didn't deserve this.

I started to go to Families Anonymous, and I saw pretty quickly that there were a lot of people there like me. I was less isolated, and this made an immediate difference to how I felt about myself. We were all struggling with things.

Some of the people at FA knew a lot more about the disease, and that we didn't cause it, we can't control it, and we can't cure it. I began to stop beating myself up so much. I began to know peace and understand serenity when I understood more about addiction. I learned how to help my son by letting him take more responsibility for his choices rather than taking him off the hook and blaming myself. I also stopped focusing on feeling sorry for myself. I started to reach out to other parents who were struggling.

I also stopped being ashamed for a disease that I didn't cause in the first place. When I first started in recovery, I didn't want anyone to know that I went to FA, and I was really into the anonymity thing. Now I know that there is nothing to be ashamed of, and being open is a way to help other parents.

I can get better for myself and our son has his own choices. Recovery does happen for parents if you work on it. It's a whole new way of thinking about yourself and your situation.

· · · · ·

The promise that I relate to the most after several years in recovery is the one about how we will suddenly realize that God is doing for us what we could not do for ourselves.

I always thought that I had a close relationship with a Higher Power, but it was really at arms' length until I started working on my own recovery, my own codependency. I was in a lot of pain when I started with the First Step and really admitted to myself that my whole life was unmanageable because I had tried to control my son's drug use. I felt lost, hopeless, a lot of darkness. But then I went to Step Two, that a Power greater than myself could restore me to sanity. I started to feel hope, that I could be sane. When I went to Step Three, I wanted to surrender my will. I was ready for a new kind of relationship with a Higher Power.

In the old days, I left my Higher Power when things were going bad. It was like, "How could this be happening to me? Why was God doing this to me? How could this happen when I have been a good person?" I was mad, sort of like Job in the Bible or like in those psalms where people complain, or even Christ on the cross when he says, "Why have you forsaken me?"

I got hope back with my Twelve Step program through how it helped me develop a new relationship with my Higher Power. I realized that God was there all along, I just hadn't asked for strength to get through my situation. It made a big difference when I prayed for this strength and not for the outcome of what I wanted God to do.

I started to notice other people in FA who were there to help me, and I remembered someone saying that God speaks through people. I saw that these new FA friends were smiling, even though their kids were still abusing drugs or were dependent and out there killing themselves. These FA members were setting goals for themselves, for their own lives. I was amazed. They also encouraged me in my own growth and I started feeling much better. I had this profound feeling of spiritual gratitude for how my life was improving. This really surprised me because my son was still using, the way he is today. This is his choice, however. I have my own life.

· · · · ·

The promise I relate to the most is that we won't regret the past, nor wish to shut the door on it. I have seen it come true in my life in ways I never would have imagined when I started to follow the structure of my Twelve Step program in Families Anonymous about two years ago.

Regretting the past brings a lot of things to mind for me. First of all, I am a stepparent to my addict son. I separated myself from him a long time because I was his stepfather, even though I raised him since he was five years old, and his father wasn't around.

Someone at an FA meeting finally asked me why I kept calling him my stepson when he was 16, even though I had been his father for eleven years. He told me to take a look at how long I had been his father, and that maybe I was trying to distance myself as if he didn't come from me. This person challenged me to think about the commitment I had made to my wife to have a family. In distancing myself, I had interfered with that happening.

That was hard for me to look at, but it was really true. I stopped calling him my stepson, and I started to work on what a father really is. I have worked on not regretting the mistake I made, even though I am sorry about it. Acknowledging that mistake makes it possible to relate compassionately to other people who have also made mistakes.

When I hear other families talk, it hurts inside to hear their problems because I relate them to things I did, or how I felt. But I can help people more because I can understand them. There is no substitute for another person's similar experience when you are lonely in your pain. People say that I have helped them by admitting my own mistakes.

· · · · ·

The promise I relate to the most says we will not regret the past. The victory for me is that I have stopped obsessing over what I did or did not do. When we just accept the past, and remember it, we can take lessons from it. We don't miss what we can do in the here and now. I accept the past that I cannot change, and I have the courage to work on the present. I work on making the best of my current situation, and I really hold myself accountable to this. If you stay in the past all the time, you are probably in self-pity and you are missing out on what you can do in the here and now. You miss the future, too, because you are not working toward something.

Not regretting the past also frees me from the stigma of having a child that has problems. My friends in FA understand what we have gone through. They understand some of the things that we have had to do to help our son, like calling the police on him. Society judges parents very unfairly if kids are not perfect. I have learned to not be ashamed, or to judge myself or other parents.

. . . . .

My recovery program has helped me to not regret the past in terms of all the pain I have had that the child I used to know isn't here any more as a result of his drug addiction. He is out there as a practicing addict, and there have been times when I didn't know if he was dead or alive. I wanted him back desperately, and even as I talk about this, I get tears in my eyes related to that struggle.

His addiction has been a tremendous loss, and I have struggled with not even wanting to remember the wonderful times we had before he started with drugs. It was too painful to remember what was gone, and what may never come back. What I have worked on, however, is accepting my son's disease, and respecting him for what he is dealing with. That has added an even deeper love for him. I can remember the happy times with him in the past and celebrate them, not regret them. I cherish them even more by not wishing them away.

. . . . .

The promise I relate to the most is the one that says we will know how to handle situations that used to baffle us.

There are so many ways that promise has come true in my life. First of all, when I first started to go to the family and parent groups at my daughter's treatment program, I lived in fear that she would relapse, and that the lives of all of us would fall apart all over again. Our parent-group counselor kept assuring us that it wouldn't be the same if that happened, because we were changing. We were learning new skills in recovery. If we chose to use them, we wouldn't have those roller coaster rides. She was tough on us, and gave us all these handouts to read. We were also required to go to FA or Al-Anon.

I started believing that if I worked on myself, I would be prepared for whatever happened. My daughter did relapse, but I had learned about my own parenting traps and codependency. I knew how to not enable her this time. I also knew how to use court consequences, and how to go to her school to ask the principal to hold her accountable.

I also returned to a hobby I had before my life was so consumed with my daughter and started writing stories and poetry. I even went back to school to finish up a degree. I was amazed; when my daughter was using as a teenager, I had no energy.

Things are not always going well with my daughter, but I have changed. I can't even remember the last time I was on one of my roller coaster plunges. I am asked by others to help them with their recoveries, and I amaze myself that I know some of the things that I do.

I have learned how to live recovery and I am really happy about that. I am always reminded of how asking for God's help made it happen. I didn't have the answers before, and I had no confidence that I would know how to handle things in the future. I am grateful every day with how recovery has changed my life.

・ ・ ・ ・ ・

I have been the beneficiary of all the promises, but the one that says it all is about knowing a new freedom and a new happiness.

I am in both FA and AA, and I have had gratitude on so many levels. I have changed in my relationship with my son and that has given me great happiness.

Recovery has also given me greater happiness than I have ever known in my entire life, including childhood. I was always self-reliant, depending on no one, and no Higher Power of any kind. I still do not believe in a deity, but I am spiritual in my approach, even though I am not religious.

I was also so much into taking action, and no action was worse than incorrect action. Now I have learned to deal with impatience, and I have tools to help me to slow down and think before I act.

I have learned through recovery how to not act on my impulses with a lot of things, including alcohol, and my destructive ways of handling relationships. I have even been able to quit smoking using the principles of my recovery.

I will never be able to repay the benefits I have received from Twelve Step recovery. It has given me a way of dealing with life that I never would have gotten otherwise.

$$\cdot \ \cdot \ \cdot \ \cdot \ \cdot$$

I have received benefits from all of the Twelve Steps, the slogans, and the Serenity Prayer. The promises that mean the most to me are the ones about comprehending the word "serenity" and knowing peace.

I am one of those who say that I am glad that my addict child brought me to recovery. Without him, without all the problems he had, I would not have walked in the door. Today, the quality of life that I want would not survive without living a recovery program.

I look back over my life and all the problems I had, and there were many signs that I needed to work on myself. It wasn't until I was hit by a two-by-four through my son's troubles, and my codependent response to them, that I realized how much I needed to work on myself.

My peace and serenity started in the couple of hours every week when my wife and I would go to a Families Anonymous meeting. It was a wonderful release to be with other parents who understood, and to get their experience, strength, and help.

The peace was also because we knew that we were going to be okay, and that God cared about our children. I pray every day that our two addicted children will ask for God's help. Recovery is there for them if they ask. It is there for all of us.

Taking care of yourself

This chapter encourages all parents who are dealing with their teenagers' substance abuse and addiction/alcoholism. The preceding ten chapters describe what to do in order to get to the point where you feel empowered. As parents say in recovery, "It works if you work it." The parents speaking in these eleven chapters are cheering you on!

Resources

VARIOUS CHAPTERS POINTED the way to this section, and material referenced is listed. In addition, the books and other resources listed here can help you explore material discussed in the chapters on a deeper level. Certain resources are also annotated.

The list is intended to be helpful, but it is not exhaustive. Books and journal articles have resource sections of their own that will contain other listings. You will also find other related titles in your library or bookstore when you look for these.

Use, abuse, dependency, assessment, and treatment

Books

American Psychiatric Association. *Diagnostic and Statistical Manual of Mental Disorders, Fourth Edition* (DSM-IV). Washington, DC: 1994.

Crowley, James. *Alliance for Change: A Plan for Community Action on Adolescent Drug Abuse*. Minneapolis: Community Intervention, Inc., 1984. A wonderful resource for understanding what communities can do to help young people. Specific ideas given can be helpful in planning. Community Intervention has other materials as well and offers training. Call (800) 328-0417.

Johnson, Vernon E., DD. *Everything You Need to Know About Chemical Dependence*. Minneapolis: The Johnson Institute, 1990. The title says it all!

Johnson, Vernon E., DD. *I'll Quit Tomorrow*. San Francisco: Harper and Row, 1980. A classic in the field. This book gives a clear understanding of how denial, delusion, and rationalization work for the addict.

Johnson, Vernon E., DD. *Intervention: How to Help Someone Who Doesn't Want Help*. Minneapolis: The Johnson Institute, 1986. The intervention procedure is powerful in helping addicts to get to treatment. This book describes this process in easy terms.

Keene, Nancy. *Working with Your Doctor: Getting the Healthcare You Deserve*. Sebastopol, CA: O'Reilly & Associates, Inc., 1998. A wonderful book to have in the home library.

Mooney, Al J., Arlene Eisenberg, and Howard Eisenberg. *The Recovery Book*. New York: Workman Publishing, 1992. A comprehensive, well-written guide to recovery, especially for the addict/alcoholic.

Schuckit, Marc A., MD. *Drug and Alcohol Abuse: A Clinical Guide to Diagnosis and Treatment*. New York: Plenum, 1995. More scholarly, but very comprehensive.

Thomas, Alexander, and Stella Chess. *Temperament and Development*. New York: Bruner/Mazel, 1977. This is the classic book on this fascinating subject.

Magazine or journal articles

Beitchman, J.H., et al. "Adolescent substance use disorders: Findings from a four-teen-year follow-up of speech/language impaired and control children." *Journal of Clinical Child Psychology* 28, no. 3 (1999): 312-21. Joseph Beitchman, MD, is a leader in this field in Canada. The article is fascinating.

Kessler, R.C., et al. "The epidemiology of co-occurring addictive and mental disorders: Implications for prevention and service utilization." *American Journal of Orthopsychiatry* 66 (1966): 17-31. Especially helpful for practitioners.

Nash, Madeleine. "How We Get Addicted and How We Might Get Cured." *Time*, 7 May 1997, 69-76.

Weinberg, N.Z., et al. "Adolescent substance abuse: A review of the past ten years." *Journal of the American Academy of Adolescent Psychiatry* 37 (1998): 252-61. This comprehensive article documents 93 other journal articles in its references for those interested in a clinical review of the literature.

Adolescent treatment programs

Chapter 4, *Treatment/Rehabilitation*, describes how to find a quality treatment program. Many of these exist all over the United States and Canada. Quality adolescent treatment will involve ongoing family treatment, but programs do exist where you take your child out of your area and return for an intense family week. The ideal is to find a program locally where you commute several times a week for family treatment and a parent education/support group.

If you are looking for treatment in the United States or Canada, or are willing to travel to Minnesota to place your child and to return for a week of family treatment, Hazelden is a resource:

Hazelden Foundation
PO Box 11
15245 Pleasant Valley Road
Center City, Minnesota 55012
(800) 833-4497

Center for youth and families.

Canadian harm reduction model

Books

Keene, Jan. *Drug Misuse: Prevention, Harm Minimisation, and Treatment*. London: Chapman and Hall, 1997. HV 5840 G7 K44 1997.

Plant, Martin A., Eric Single, and Tim Stockwell. *Alcohol: Minimising the Harm: What Works?* London: Free Association Books, 1997. HV 5035 .A45645 1997.

Single, Eric. *Harm Reduction, Drugs and Alcohol: Future Directions*. Ottawa: Canadian Centre on Substance Abuse, 1995. HV 5801 .S525 1995.

Internet resources

CCSA (Canadian Centre on Substance Abuse)
http://www.ccsa.ca/

CEIDA (Centre for Education and Information on Drugs and Alcohol)
http://www.ceida.net.au/

Lindesmith Center
http://www.lindesmith.org/

NAMA (National Alliance of Methadone Advocates)
http://www.methadone.org/

Adolescence

Books

Blos, Peter. *The Adolescent Passage: Developmental Issues.* New York: International Universities, 1979. A helpful overview. This author has a wide reputation for being scholarly yet readable.

Caldwell, Elizabeth. *Teenagers: A Bewildered Parent's Guide.* San Diego: Silvercat, 1996. Easy and informative.

Esman, Aaron, editor. *The Psychology of Adolescence.* New York: International Universities, 1975. A fascinating collection of writings from a wide range of individuals who have written about this age group.

Hersch, Patricia. *A Tribe Apart: A Journey into the Heart of American Adolescence.* New York: Ballantine, 1999. Author studied eight teenagers in Virginia for three years and describes this age group well.

King, Stephen. *Christine.* New York: Viking, 1983. A typical Steven King supernatural horror novel, but it is one of the best pieces of writing about what it is like to be a misfit, lonely teenager. The inner workings of the teenage mind are described better than you will ever get in a psychology book.

Piffer, Mary. *The Shelter of Each Other: Rebuilding Our Families.* New York: Random House, 1996. Particularly good on the pressures of adolescence facing young women.

Weiner, Irving. *Psychological Disturbance in Adolescence.* New York: John Wiley, 1970. A classic. Many scholarly references.

Magazines

Gibbs, Nancy. "A Week in the Life of a High School: What It's Really Like Since Columbine." *Time,* 25 Oct 1999, 66-115. The author and a team of writers describe a week in Webster Groves High School in Missouri. Detailed and fascinating. A great awareness of contemporary teen culture.

Newsweek, 3 May 1999, 22-39. The cover on this issue asks "Why?" and various articles explore the Littleton massacre and the science of teen violence.

"The Secret Life of Teens." *Newsweek*, 10 May 1999, 36-59. There are a series of articles describing teens in this issue that are a must-read for those trying to understand this age group.

Newspapers

Call your local high school and ask for the last three copies of the school newspaper. This is a helpful way to see what goes on in the school culture that is so much of an adolescent's day.

Feelings, communication, stress, and codependency issues

Books

Beattie, Melody. *Beyond Codependency and Getting Better All the Time*. San Francisco: Harper/Hazelden, 1989. A helpful guide on how to get better. Beattie has many titles to explore.

Benson, Herbert. *The Relaxation Response*. New York: Avon Books, 1975. This number one best seller is the classic in stress reduction techniques. A wonderful listing of supplemental resources at the end.

Black, Claudia. *Repeat After Me*. Denver: MAC Printing and Publication, 1985. A workbook to help you work on your own issues.

Breathnach, Sarah Ban. *Simple Abundance: A Daybook of Comfort and Joy*. NewYork: Warner Books, 1995. An affirming book of daily readings to help you encourage yourself. Breathnach has a whole line of related books. Check out other titles as well.

Buscaglia, Leo. *Loving Each other: The Challenge of Human Relationships*. Thorofare, New Jersey: Slack, 1984. A gentle guide.

Edelman, Hope, ed. *Letters from Motherless Daughters: Words of Courage, Grief, and Healing*. New York: Addison Wesley, 1999. A companion book to the book below, with letters from women who read the first book.

Edelman, Hope. *Motherless Daughters: The Legacy of Loss*. New York: Addison Wesley, 1994. A wonderful book for women who are exploring the impact of this loss on their lives.

Ellis, Albert, and Robert Harper. *A New Guide to Rational Living*. North Hollywood, CA: Wilshire Books, 1977. A helpful book that shows how the messages we give to ourselves can be interrupted.

Fossum, Merle. *Catching Fire: Men Coming Alive in Recovery*. San Francisco: Harper/Hazelden, 1989. Especially helpful for men.

Friedman, Sonya. *On a Clear Day You Can See Yourself*. New York: Ivy Books, 1991. A nurturing, affirming book for women that helps you look honestly at destructive ways you think and act that only make you more miserable.

Gibbons, Kaye. *Sights Unseen*. New York: G.P. Putnam's Sons, 1995. An excellent novel about growing up with a mentally ill parent. It was written by the author of *Ellen Foster*, another good book about growing up with alcoholism. *Ellen Foster* was made into a television movie, so you might be able to find it at your video store. Look at all of the books by this author. There may be additional titles that will speak to you.

Gordon, Barry. *Your Father, Your Self: How Sons and Daughters Can Understand and Heal Their Relationships with Their Fathers*. Secaucus: Carol Communications, 1996. A wonderful book even if you do not think you have anything to heal. The author helps you to think about this relationship and how you may be perpetuating patterns with your own children that did not work well when you were growing up.

Keyes, Ralph, ed. *Sons on Fathers: A Book of Men's Writing*. New York: HarperCollins, 1992. A wonderful book for men that shares a variety of common experiences.

Lunden, Joan. *A Bend in the Road Is Not the End of the Road*. New York: William Morrow, 1998. An affirming, enthusiastic book to help you in your desire to grow.

McKay, Gary, and Don C. Dinkmeyer. *How You Feel Is Up to You: The Power of Emotional Choice*. San Luis Obispo, CA: Impact, 1994. Helps you with choices you can make to be healthier.

McFarland, Barbara, and Tyeis Baker-Baumann. *Feeding the Empty Heart: Adult Children and Compulsive Eating*. Center City, Minnesota: Hazelden, 1988. Helps you explore how eating may be a result of stress and what to do about it.

Naparstek, Belleruth. *Your Sixth Sense: Activating Your Psychic Potential*. New York: HarperCollins, 1997. Reinforces the importance of trusting your intuition.

Napier, Augustus, and Carl Whitaker. *The Family Crucible*. New York: Harper and Row, 1978. A classic in the field of family therapy.

SARK. *Succulent Wild Woman*. New York: Fireside, 1997. Especially good if you are trying to encourage a new you.

SARK. *The Bodacious Book of Succulence*. New York: Simon and Schuster/Fireside, 1998. Women who have not discovered this author are missing something. Every book she writes is wonderful.

Taylor, Elizabeth. *Elizabeth Takes Off*. New York: Putnam, 1987. An inspiring book on how to improve your self-esteem and not engage in compulsive eating to deal with stress.

Vanzant, Iyanla. *Don't Give It Away: A Workbook of Self-Awareness and Self-Affirmations for Young Women*. New York: Fireside, 1999. This author has many wonderful titles. This is an empowering workbook for women of any age.

Vanzant, Iyanla. *The Value in the Valley: A Black Woman's Guide Through Life's Dilemmas*. A wonderful book for any woman. Filled with support and guidance to handle many challenges.

Viorst, Judith. *Imperfect Control: Our Lifelong Struggles with Power and Surrender*. New York: Simon and Schuster/Fireside, 1998. A wonderful book to encourage you to change and give up what is not working for you.

Viorst, Judith. *Necessary Losses: The Loves, Illusions, Dependencies, and Impossible Expectations that All of Us Have to Give Up in Order to Grow*. New York: Simon and Schuster, 1986. Especially good in facing the reality of what we have to give up.

Wegscheider-Cruse, Sharon. *Another Chance: Hope and Health for the Alcoholic Family*. Palo Alto, CA: Science and Behavior Books, Inc., 1981. A classic in understanding families struggling with alcoholism.

Whitfield, Charles. *Co-Dependence: Healing the Human Condition*. Deerfield Beach, FL: Health Communications, 1991. An overview of the condition and what to do to heal.

Films to explore feelings

The following movies are recommended:

Before and After
> Shows the codependent lengths parents will go to help their child, and the consequences of this. Based on the book by Rosellen Brown. A gripping story. With Meryl Streep and Liam Neeson.

Blue Sky
> Deals with growing up with a manic-depressive parent or any parent who has mood swings.

Frances
> Deals with growing up with a severely mentally ill parent.

Prince of Tides
> Deals with growing up in an alcoholic home.

Tender Mercies
> Deals with growing up in an abusive home.

The Burning Bed
> Deals with growing up in an abusive home.

The Great Santini
> Deals with growing up in an alcoholic home.

Recordings to explore feelings

Seek out recordings that have emotion. Some recommended composers for this process are Wagner, Tchaikovsky, Beethoven (in particular the Fifth and the Ninth Symphonies), and Mozart (Don Giovanni opera, parts of which are on the soundtrack of the film *Amadeus*).

Many parents report that recording artists such as Bette Midler, Barbra Streisand, Celine Dion, and even Madonna (her post-childbirth songs) speak to them deeply in the well of feelings. Roberta Flack is also recommended, particularly CDs that have a collection of her greatest hits, including "The First Time Ever I Saw Your Face" and "That's No Way to Say Goodbye."

With whatever music you choose, it is important to dive in and experience the words, the orchestration, and so on. You want to immerse yourself and see what happens.

Also, check out Nature Solitude CDs or tapes when you go to a large bookstore. You can be on a nature walk while you are in the car, doing housework, or when you have locked yourself in the bathroom to read your Al-Anon or Families Anonymous material.

Representative sample of codependency treatment programs

Betty Ford Center
39000 Bob Hope Drive
Rancho Mirage, California 92270
(800) 854-9211

Call to request a video if you want to see the location and get more information. In addition to many fine alcohol/drug treatment programs, the Betty Ford Center has an intensive outpatient program for codependency issues. This is a four-day program and is called a workshop. It is offered every three to four months. Those attending stay at a local hotel. There is also a six-week outpatient program for those who can commute.

Hazelden Foundation
PO Box 11
15245 Pleasant Valley Road
Center City, Minnesota 55012
(800) 257-7800

Call to request a video of the location and other information. In addition to many fine alcohol/drug treatment programs, Hazelden has a five- to seven-day codependency/family issues program. Participants live on-site, but it is also possible to commute.

Mind/Body Institute
5124 Mayfield Road #258
Lyndhurst/Cleveland, Ohio 44124
(216) 831-7412

Call or write for services and to request reprints of articles, speeches, reading list, and brochure, or to speak with Gary Gottlieb, MD, president. Look for programs like this in your own community.

On-Site
10 Court Square
Charlotte, Tennessee 37036
(800) 341-7432

On-Site offers a number of very creative workshops on an outpatient basis for those who can commute. They also offer an intensive residential program for codependency issues where participants live on the campus for six or seven days.

Sierra Tucson
39580 South Lago Del Oro Parkway
Tucson, Arizona 85739
(800) 854-9211

Call to request a video to see the location. Sierra Tucson offers a 26–30 day residential program, no outpatient programs.

Working on recovery, empowerment

All three of the following books are helpful guides to the basics of Al-Anon:

Al-Anon Faces Alcoholism. New York: Al-Anon Family Group Headquarters, 1984.

Al-Anon Family Groups. New York: Al-Anon Family Group Headquarters, 1984.

Al-Anon's Twelve Steps and Twelve Traditions. New York: Al-Anon Family Group Headquarters, 1987.

Also helpful are:

Alcoholics Anonymous: The Story of How Many Thousands of Men and Women Have Recovered from Alcoholism, Third Edition. New York: Alcoholics Anonymous World Services, 1976. Formal name for *The Big Book* that is the cornerstone of AA. The founders wrote it.

Dr. Bob and the Good Old-timers. New York: Alcoholics Anonymous World Services, 1980. Fascinating biography of one of the founders of AA, with recollections of early AA in the Midwest.

Ford, Betty, with Chris Chase. *The Times of My Life*. New York: Harper and Row, 1978. An inspiring biography of an inspiring woman.

Hemfelt, Robert, PhD, and Richard Fowler, PhD. *Serenity: A Companion Guide for Twelve-Step Recovery*. Nashville: Thomas Nelson Publishers, 1990. Matches biblical scripture to recovery. It is a helpful supplement for Christians wanting to deepen recovery with biblical support.

Kurtz, Ernest. *Not God: A History of Alcoholics Anonymous*. Center City, MN: Hazelden, 1979. A comprehensive history of AA, debates within about philosophy and structure, how it spread, and so on.

Larsen, Earnie. *Stage II Recovery: Life Beyond Addiction*. Minneapolis: Winston Press, 1985. A readable book with many ideas for alcoholics about later recovery.

McGovern, George. *Terry: My Daughter's Life-and-Death Struggle with Alcoholism*. New York: Penguin/Plume, 1997. A deeply felt description of how alcoholism works, written by a popular Senator and Presidential candidate.

Mooney, Al J., Arlene Eisenberg, and Howard Eisenberg. *The Recovery Book*. New York: Workman Publishing, 1992. A comprehensive, clear, and highly readable source for every recovering family.

The Twelve Steps for Everyone …who really wants them. Minneapolis: Comp Care, 1975. Helpful and enriching descriptions of what the Steps mean.

Working on letting go

Halberstam, Yitta, and Judith Leventhal. *Small Miracles: Extraordinary Coincidences from Everyday Life*. Holbrook, MA: Adams Media, 1997. A wonderful book of short essays describing true experiences that help us remember the possibilities and blessings in our lives.

Kaufman, Barry Neil. *Happiness Is a Choice*. New York: Ballantine/Fawcett Columbine, 1991. Things we need to let go of if we are going to be happy.

Kushner, Harold. *When All You've Ever Wanted Isn't Enough: The Search for a Life That Matters*. New York: Summit Books, 1986. Rabbi Kushner speaks on profound levels about how to improve our lives.

Peck, M. Scott. *The Road Less Traveled: A New Psychology of Love, Traditional Values, and Spiritual Growth*. New York: Simon & Schuster, 1978. A widely read book. There are even discussion groups available with study guides to explore the material. Check with your local bookstore about how to access these or how to find the guide and start your own discussion group.

Twerski, Abraham, MD. *Caution: Kindness Can Be Dangerous to the Alcoholic*. Englewood Cliffs, NJ: Prentice-Hall, 1981. This title is often quoted as one of the best descriptions of what is needed to help an addict/alcoholic. Twerski is a rabbi/physician who leads workshops and is one of the best speakers around. This book is out of print, but can be found in used bookstores.

Providing natural consequences

Faber, Adele, and Elaine Mazlish. *How to Talk So Kids Can Learn.* New York: Fireside, 1995. Directed to help kids learn at school, but principles can also be applied at home.

Faber, Adele, and Elaine Mazlish. *How to Talk So Kids Will Listen and Listen So Kids Will Talk.* New York: Avon, 1980. The title says it all. Helpful in avoiding power struggles.

Faber, Adele, and Elaine Mazlish. *Liberated Parents, Liberated Children: Your Guide to a Happier Family.* New York: Avon, 1990. Based on the theories of Dr. Haim Ginott. Helps parents deal respectfully with children.

Glasser, Naomi, ed. *Control Theory in the Practice of Reality Therapy.* New York: Harper and Row, 1989. Essays from practitioners who applied reality therapy. A good overview of how it works.

Glasser, William. *Reality Therapy.* New York: Harper and Row, 1965. Basic theories made very readable. Second half of book deals with application at Ventura with severely delinquent adolescent girls.

Glasser, William. *Schools Without Failure.* New York: Harper and Row, 1969. Title says it all. Ideas can be applied in treatment programs and at home.

Glasser, William. *The Quality School: Managing Students Without Coercion.* New York: Harper and Row, 1990. Same as above title.

Nelsen, Jane, and Lynn Lott. *Positive Discipline for Teenagers.* Rocklin, CA: Prima, 1994. Ways to sidestep conflict and work together.

Nolte, Dorothy Law, and Rachel Harris. *Children Learn What They Live.* New York: Workman, 1998. Good reminder of how parents' actions speak louder than words and how to build positive self esteem in children.

Schofield, Deniece. *Confessions of a Happily Organized Family.* Cincinnati: Writers Digest, 1984. Great ideas on how to organize better.

Wubbolding, Robert E. *Using Reality Therapy.* New York: Harper and Row, 1988. Implementing reality therapy techniques.

Information and Help

INFORMATION BELOW is organized into three main topics: support groups, counseling referrals, and information on drug prevention and treatment. Special thanks to the US Department of Education for some of this information, which can be found in English and Spanish in the booklet *Growing Up Drug-Free: A Parent's Guide to Prevention*. Free copies are available by calling (877) 4ED-PUBS.

Support groups

Al-Anon/Alateen Family Group Headquarters
1600 Corporate Landing Parkway
Virginia Beech, VA 23454-5617
(800) 344-2666 or (800) 356-9996
http://www.al-anon.alateen.org/

Alcoholics Anonymous World Services
475 Riverside Drive
New York, NY 10115
(212) 870-3400
http://www.aa.org/

A worldwide fellowship of sober alcoholics whose recovery is based on Twelve Steps. No dues or fees; self-supporting through small voluntary member contributions. Accepts no outside funds; not affiliated with any other organization.

Families Anonymous, Inc.
PO Box 3475
Culver City, CA 90231-3475
(800) 736-9805 or (310) 313-5800
http://www.familiesanonymous.org/

Nar-Anon Family Group Headquarters
PO Box 2562
Palos Verdes Peninsula, CA 90274-8562
(310) 547-5800

Narcotics Anonymous
PO Box 9999
Van Nuys, CA 91409-9099
(818) 773-9999
http://www.wsoinc.com/

Toughlove International
PO Box 1069
Doylestown, PA 18901
(800) 333-1069
http://www.toughlove.org/

Counseling referrals

American Academy of Child and Adolescent Psychiatry
(202) 966-7300
http://www.aacap.org/

American Counseling Association
(800) 347-6647
http://www.counseling.org/

American Psychiatric Association
(202) 682-6000
http://www.psych.org/

American Psychological Association
(800) 964-2000
http://www.apa.org/

National Alliance for the Mentally Ill
(800) 950-6264
http://www.nami.org/

National Association of Social Workers
(800) 638-8799
http://www.naswdc.org/

National Board for Certified Counselors
(910) 547-0607
http://www.nbcc.org/

National Mental Health Association
(800) 969-6642
http://www.nmha.org/

Advocates advise consumers to ask mental health professionals about their education, credentials, areas of specialty, and the type of treatment they provide. Many find it takes a while to find a therapist who suits them.

The best resource is to ask others whom they have used.

Information on drug prevention and treatment

African American Family Services (AAFS)
2616 Nicollet Avenue
Minneapolis, MN 55408
(612) 871-7878 or (800) 557-2180
http://www.aafs-mn.org/

American Cancer Society
1599 Clifton Road, NE
Atlanta, GA 30329
(800) 227-2345
http://www.cancer.org/

American Council for Drug Education
164 W. 74th Street
New York, NY 10023
Information: (800) 488-DRUG, *http://www.acde.org/*
Referrals: (800) DRUG-HEL (P), *http://www.drughelp.org/*
For immediate specific assistance or referral:
(800) COCAINE
(888) MARIJUA (NA)
(800) HELP111
(800) 9HEROIN
(800) RELAPSE
(800) CRISIS9

CDC National AIDS Clearinghouse
(CDC National Prevention Information Network)
PO Box 6003
Rockville, MD 20849-6003
(800) 458-5231
http://www.cdcnpin.org/

Department of Health and Human Services
Washington, DC
(800) 729-6686

Request catalogue called *National Directory of Drug Abuse and Alcohol Treatment and Prevention* if this is not in your library.

Hazelden Foundation
PO Box 176
Center City, MN 55012-1076
(800) 257-7800
http://www.hazelden.com/

Join Together
441 Stuart Street, 7th Floor
Boston, MA 02116
(617) 437-1500
http://www.jointogether.org/

National Council on Alcoholism and Drug Dependence, Inc.
12 W. 21st Street, 7th Floor
New York, NY 10010
(212) 206-6770 or (800) NCA-CALL
http://www.ncadd.org/

National Crime Prevention Council
PO Box 1
100 Church Street
Amsterdam, NY 12010
(800) 627-2911
http://www.ncpc.org/

National Institute on Drug Abuse
5600 Fishers Lane
Rockville, MD 20857
(301) 443-1124
http://www.nida.nih.gov/

National PTA Drug and Alcohol Abuse Prevention Project
330 North Wabash Avenue, Suite 2100
Chicago, IL 60611-3690
(800) 307-4782 or (312) 670-6782
http://www.pta.org/

Parent to Parent
1240 Johnson Ferry Place, Suite F10
Marietta, GA 30068
(800) 487-7743

Parents and Adolescents Recovering Together Successfully (PARTS)
12815 Stebick Court
San Diego, CA 92310-2705
(619) 698-3449

Partnership for a Drug-Free America
405 Lexington Avenue, Suite 1601
New York, NY 10174
(212) 922-1560
http://www.drugfreeamerica.org/

Safe and Drug-Free Schools
US Department of Education
400 Maryland Avenue, SW
Washington, DC 20202-6123
(202) 260-3954
Publications: (877) 433-7827
http://www.ed.gov/offices/OESE/SDFS/

SafeHomes
c/o Erie County Council for the Prevention of Alcohol and Substance Abuse
4255 Harlem Road
Amherst, NY 14226
(716) 839-1157

**Substance Abuse and Mental Health Services Administration (SAMHSA)/
Center for Substance Abuse Treatment (CSAT)**
NCADI
PO Box 2345
Rockville, MD 20847-2345
(800) 662-HELP
http://www.drughelp.org/

**Substance Abuse and Mental Health Services Administration (SAMHSA)/
National Clearinghouse for Alcohol and Drug Information (NCADI)**
PO Box 2345
Rockville, MD 20847-2345
(800) SAY-NOTO
http://www.health.org/

Youth Power
2000 Franklin Street, Suite 400
Oakland, CA 94612
(510) 451-6666 or (800) 258-2766
http://www.youthpower.org/

Specific Drugs and Their Effects

ADOLESCENTS USE MANY DRUGS that are known by a variety of names. The list below gives generic names and street names as well as how the drugs are consumed, their effects, and helpful facts for parents. Special thanks to the US Department of Education for abbreviated information, which can be found in English and Spanish in the booklet *Growing Up Drug-Free: A Parent's Guide to Prevention*. Free copies are available by calling (877) 4ED-PUBS.

Depressants

Alcohol

Other names: Beer, wine, liquor, cooler, malt liquor, booze. Alcohol is often identified by how it is sold, and adolescents use terms like forty, quarts, and cheap quarts.

How consumed: Orally.

Effects: Addiction (alcoholism), dizziness, slurred speech, disturbed sleep, nausea, vomiting, hangovers, impaired motor skills, violent behavior, impaired learning, fetal alcohol syndrome, respiratory depression, death (with high doses).

Facts for parents: Twenty-five percent of eighth-graders have admitted to being intoxicated at least once. Adolescents can often mix alcohol in fruit drinks, mouthwash, and Kool-Aid containers. Binge drinking is a major health concern for teenagers because high alcohol levels cause the brain to shut down respiration. Alcohol poisoning, and death, is the result.

Stimulants

Amphetamines

Other names: Speed, uppers, ups, hearts, black beauties, pep pills, copilots, bumble bees, Benzedrine, Dexedrine, footballs, biphetamines.

How consumed: Orally, injected, snorted, or smoked.

Effects: Addiction, irritability, anxiety, increased blood pressure, paranoia, psychosis, depression, aggression, convulsions, dilated pupils and blurred vision, dizziness, sleeplessness, loss of appetite, malnutrition, increased body temperature, increased risk of exposure to HIV, hepatitis, and other infectious diseases if injected.

Facts for parents: Chronic use can induce psychosis with symptoms similar to schizophrenia, i.e., paranoia, visual and auditory hallucinations.

Cocaine

Other names: Coke, snow, nose candy, flake, blow, big C, lady, girl, white, snowbirds.

How consumed: Snorted or dissolved in water and injected. When laced (sprinkled) on marijuana, the combination is called blunt.

Effects: Addiction, pupil dilation, elevated blood pressure and heart rate, increased respiratory rate, increased risk of exposure to HIV, hepatitis, and other infectious diseases if injected, paranoia, seizures, heart attack, respiratory failure, constricted peripheral blood vessels, restlessness, irritability, anxiety, loss of appetite, tactile hallucinations, insomnia, increased body temperature, death from overdose.

Facts for parents: Cocaine is a powerfully addictive drug. Heavy use may produce hallucinations, paranoia, aggression, insomnia, and depression.

Crack

Other names: Rock, freebase, bump, stones.

How consumed: Heated and smoked in a pipe. When laced (sprinkled) on marijuana, the combination is called blunt.

Effects: Addiction, pupil dilation, elevated blood pressure and heart rate, increased respiratory rate, increased risk of exposure to HIV, hepatitis, and other infectious diseases if injected, paranoia, seizures, heart attack, respiratory failure, constricted peripheral blood vessels, restlessness, irritability, anxiety, loss of appetite, tactile hallucinations, insomnia, increased body temperature, death from overdose.

Facts for parents: A cheaper form of cocaine that may be more addicting.

Designer drugs (fentanyl-based)

Other names: Synthetic heroin, goodfella.

How consumed: Injected, sniffed, or smoked.

Effects: Instant respiratory paralysis, potency creates strong possibility for overdose, increased risk of exposure to HIV, hepatitis, and other infectious diseases if injected, many of the same effects as heroin.

Facts for parents: Changing the molecular structure of an existing drug or drugs to create a new substance creates designer drugs.

Ecstasy (methylenedioxy amphetamine)

Other names: X, XTC, Adam, MDMA, rolls, XYC.

How consumed: Orally.

Effects: Psychiatric disturbances including panic, anxiety, depression, and paranoia, muscle tension, nausea, blurred vision, sweating, increased heart rate and blood pressure, tremors, hallucinations, reduced appetite, sleep problems, fainting, chills.

Facts for parents: Ecstasy is popular at all-night underground dance parties (called "raves") and is the most common "designer drug." It is a major, rising drug for adolescents. It can be put in drinks without others detecting it before it is too late. Users tend to carry water with them because it causes dehydration.

GHB (gamma hydroxybutyic acid)

Other names: Liquid ecstasy, somatomax, scoop, grievous bodily harm, liquid x, Georgia home boy, goop.

How consumed: Snorted, orally in liquid form, smoked, or mixed into drinks.

Effects: Liver failure, vomiting, tremors, seizures, comas, fatal respiratory problems.

Facts for parents: Sometimes the user transports the drug in empty hotel shampoo or eyedropper bottles.

Herbal ecstasy/ephedrine

Other names: Herbal ecstasy, cloud 9, rave energy, ultimate Xphoria, X, XYC, XTC.

How consumed: Orally.

Effects: Increased heart rate and blood pressure, seizures, heart attacks, stroke, death.

Facts for parents: The active ingredients in Herbal Ecstasy are caffeine and ephedrine.

Methamphetamine

Other names: Speed, meth, crank, crystal, ice, fire, croak, crypto, white cross, glass.

How consumed: Orally, injected, snorted, or smoked.

Effects: Addiction, irritability, anxiety, increased blood pressure, paranoia/psychosis, aggression, nervousness, hyperthermia, compulsive behavior, stroke, depression, convulsions, heart and blood vessel toxicity, insomnia, loss of appetite, malnutrition, hallucinations, increased sexual desires, the sensation of insects creeping on or under the skin, arrhythmia, increased risk of exposure to HIV, hepatitis, and other infectious diseases if injected.

Facts for parents: Some users avoid sleep for three to fifteen days. "Ice" is the street name for smokable methamphetamine.

Ritalin (methylphenidate)

Other names: Speed, west coast.

How consumed: Tablet is crushed, and the powder is snorted or injected.

Effects: Loss of appetite, fevers, convulsions, severe headaches, increased risk of exposure to HIV, hepatitis, and other infectious diseases if injected, irregular heartbeat and respiration, paranoia, hallucinations, delusions, excessive repetition of movements and meaningless tasks, tremors, muscle twitching.

Facts for parents: Ritalin, a legally prescribed medication for treating attention deficit disorder and hyperactivity, is sometimes sold and abused as a street drug. Some children buy or steal the drug from their classmates.

Opiates/opiate-like

Heroin

Other names: Smack, horse, mud, brown sugar, junk, black tar, big H, dope, dog food.

How consumed: Injected, smoked, or snorted.

Effects: Addiction, slowed and slurred speech, slow gait, constricted pupils, droopy eyelids, impaired night vision, vomiting after first use and at very high doses, decreased sexual pleasure, indifference to sex, reduced appetite, constipation, nodding off (at high doses), respiratory depression or failure, increased risk of exposure to HIV, hepatitis, and other infectious diseases if injected, dry, itching skin and skin infections, death from overdose.

Facts for parents: Heroin users quickly develop a tolerance to the drug and need more and more of it to get the same effects or even to feel well.

Rohypnol (flunitrazepam)

Other names: Roach, roofies, the forget pill, rope, rophies, ruffies, R2, roofenol, la roche, rib.

How consumed: Orally in pill form, dissolved in a drink, or snorted.

Effects: Addiction, blackouts with a complete loss of memory, a sense of fearlessness and aggression, dizziness and disorientation, nausea, difficulty with motor movements and speaking.

Facts for parents: Referred to as the "date-rape" drug. Creates a drunken feeling that lasts two to eight hours.

"Special K" (ketamine hydrochloride)

Other names: Vitamin K, new ecstasy, psychedelic heroin, ketalar, ketaject, super-K, breakfast cereal.

How consumed: Snorted or smoked.

Effects: Delirium, amnesia, impaired motor function, potentially fatal respiratory problems.

Facts for parents: Popular at raves. Used as an anesthetic for animals.

Hallucinogens

LSD (lysergic acid diethylamide)

Other names: Acid, microdot, tabs, doses, trips, hits, sugar cubes, L.

How consumed: Tabs taken orally or gelatin/liquid put in eyes.

Effects: Elevated body temperature and blood pressure, suppressed appetite, sleeplessness, tremors, chronic recurring hallucinations.

Facts for parents: LSD is the most common hallucinogen. LSD tabs are often decorated with colorful designs or cartoon characters.

Mushrooms (psilocybin)

Other names: Shrooms, caps, magic mushrooms, fungus, fungi.

How consumed: Eaten or brewed and drunk in tea.

Effects: Increased blood pressure, sweating, nausea, and hallucinations.

Facts for parents: Many mushroom users purchase hallucinogenic mushroom spores via mail order.

PCP (phencyclidine)

Other names: Angel dust, ozone, rocket fuel, peace pill, elephant tranquilizer, dust. When added to cigarettes or marijuana, the combination can be called water, wet, Sheba, skinny Minnie.

How consumed: Snorted, smoked, orally, or injected.

Effects: Hallucinations, "out-of-body" experiences, impaired motor coordination, inability to feel physical pain, respiratory attack, depression, anxiety, disorientation, fear, panic, paranoia, aggressive behavior and violence, increased risk of exposure to HIV, hepatitis, and other infectious diseases if injected, death.

Facts for parents: Marijuana joints can be dipped into PCP without the smoker's knowledge.

Others

Inhalants

Other names: Nitrous oxide, laughing gas, whippets, aerosol sprays, cleaning fluids, solvents.

How consumed: Vapors are inhaled.

Effects: Headache, muscle weakness, abdominal pain, severe mood swings and violent behavior, numbness and tingling of hands and feet, decrease or loss of sense of smell, nausea, nosebleeds, liver, lung, and kidney damage, dangerous chemical imbalances in the body, fatigue, lack of coordination, loss of appetite, decreases in heart and respiratory rates, hepatitis or peripheral neuropathy from long-time use.

Facts for parents: Hundreds of legal household products can be sniffed or "huffed" to get high. These include whiteout, Lysol, whipped cream aerosols, and any products with propellant. All inhalants can be toxic. Adolescents can die from inhaling so deeply that they pass out.

Marijuana/hashish

Other names: Weed, pot, reefer, grass, dope, ganja, hash, Mary Jane, sinsemilla, herb, Aunt Mary, skunk, boom, kif, gangster, chronic, 420.

How consumed: Smoked or eaten.

Effects: Bloodshot eyes, dry mouth and throat, impaired or reduced comprehension, altered sense of time; reduced ability to perform tasks requiring concentration and coordination, such as driving a car; paranoia, intense anxiety or panic attacks; altered cognition, making acquiring of new information difficult; impairments in learning, memory, perception, and judgment; difficulty speaking, listening effectively, thinking, retaining knowledge, problem solving, and forming concepts.

Facts for parents: It has a sweet smell. The average age teens first use marijuana is 14, but it is getting younger every day. Marijuana can be smoked using homemade pipes and bongs made from soda cans or plastic beverage containers. Currently popular is smoking marijuana in hollowed-out cigars. Since cigar leaves are not porous, inhaling makes the marijuana even stronger and more dangerous.

Steroids

Other names: Rhoids, juice.

How consumed: Orally or injected into muscle.

Effects: Liver cancer, sterility, masculine traits in women and feminine traits in men, aggression, depression, acne, mood swings.

Facts for parents: Steroid users subject themselves to more than 70 potentially harmful side effects. Steroid abuse is on the rise for adolescents.

Tobacco

Other names: Smoke, bone, butt, coffin nail, cancer stick.

How consumed: Cigarettes, cigars, pipes, smokeless tobacco (chew, dip, snuff).

Effects: Addiction, heart and cardiovascular disease; cancer of the lung, larynx, esophagus, bladder, pancreas, kidney, and mouth; emphysema and chronic bronchitis, spontaneous abortion, pre-term delivery, and low birth weight.

Facts for parents: One in five twelfth-graders is a daily smoker.

Notes

Preface

1. Cindy Handler, *Growing Up Drug Free: A Parent's Guide to Prevention* (Washington: Partnership for a Drug-Free America, US Department of Education, 1998), 2.
2. Handler, *Growing Up Drug Free*, 2.

Chapter 1: *Use, Abuse, and Dependency*

1. Vernon E. Johnson, *Everything You Need to Know About Chemical Dependence* (Minneapolis: Johnson Institute, 1990), 13.
2. Johnson, *Everything You Need to Know About Chemical Dependence*, 13, 14.
3. S. Saul, *Chemical Dependency: An Acceptable Disease* (Center City, MN: Hazelden, 1987), 6.
4. Richard A. Knox, "On the Trail of a Pill for Alcoholism," *Cleveland Plain Dealer*, 6 Sept 1999.
5. Madeline Nash, " How We Get Addicted," *Time*, 5 May 1997, 69–76.
6. "Public Suicide Awakens City to Problem of Drug Addiction."
7. *Al-Anon's Information for the Newcomer* (Virginia: Al-Anon Family Group Headquarters). Reprinted by permission of Al-Anon Family Group Headquarters, Inc.

Chapter 2: *Patterns of Development*

1. Irving Weiner, *Psychological Disturbance in Adolescence* (New York: John Wiley, 1970), 48.
2. Stephen Hall, "The Bully in the Mirror," *New York Times Sunday Magazine*, 22 Aug 1999, 34.
3. Adrian Nicole Le Blanc, "The Outsiders," *New York Times Sunday Magazine*, 22 Aug 1999, 38.
4. Le Blanc, "The Outsiders," 38.
5. Shannon Brownlee, "Inside the Teen Brain," *US News and World Report*, 9 Aug 1999, 46–7.
6. Weiner, *Psychological Disturbance*, 48.
7. Vernon E. Johnson, *Everything You Need to Know About Chemical Dependence* (Minneapolis: The Johnson Institute, 1990), 83.
8. Jim Crowley, *Alliance for Change: A Plan for Community Action on Adolescent Drug Abuse* (Minneapolis: Community Intervention, 1984), 106–7.
9. Johnson, *Everything You Need to Know*, 84–7.
10. Crowley, 39–40.

Chapter 3: *Assessment*

1. Nancy Keene, *Working with Your Doctor* (Sebastopol, CA: O'Reilly & Associates, 1998), 29.
2. Christopher Quinn, "Punishing Youthful Offenders," *Cleveland Plain Dealer*, 18 Jul 1999, 1–7.
3. Quinn, "Punishing," 7.
4. Quinn, "Punishing," 7.
5. Judith S. Kaye, "Making the Case for Hands-On Courts," *Newsweek*, 11 Oct 1999, 13.

Chapter 4: *Treatment/Rehabilitation*

1. Al Mooney, MD, Arlene Eisenberg, and Howard Eisenberg, *The Recovery Book* (New York: Workman, 1992), 60–1.
2. Mooney, *Recovery Book*, 42–3.
3. Marc Schuckit, *Drug and Alcohol Abuse: A Clinical Guide to Diagnosis and Treatment* (New York: Plenum, 1995), 303.
4. Schuckit, *Drug and Alcohol Abuse*, 303.
5. Adolescent Provider Committee for the Alcohol and Drug Addiction Services Board of Cuyahoga County, adapt. *Managed Care Clinical Care Criteria for Placement in Different Levels of Treatment Intensity for Adolescents Presenting Psychoactive Substance Use Disorders or Who Are High Risk in Cuyahoga County* (Cleveland: 1997).

Chapter 5: *Working on Your Feelings*

1. Merle Fossum, *Catching Fire: Men Coming Alive in Their Recovery* (San Francisco: Harper/Hazelden, 1989), 21.
2. Belleruth Naparstek, *Your Sixth Sense: Activating Your Psychic Potential* (New York: Harper Collins, 1997), 49.
3. Paul Simon, "I Am a Rock," *Simon and Garfunkel's Greatest Hits*, 1972.

Chapter 6: *Harmful Consequences from Normal Feelings*

1. Sharon Weigsheider-Cruse, *Another Chance: Hope And Health for the Alcoholic Family* (Palo Alto, CA: Science and Behavior Books, 1981), 21.
2. Copyright 1983 Families Anonymous, Inc. Reprinted by permission of Families Anonymous, Inc.

Chapter 7: *Communication and Relationships*

1. Augustus Napier and Carl Whitaker, *The Family Crucible* (New York: Harper and Row, 1978), 47.

Chapter 8: *Working on Recovery*

1. *Al-Anon Family Groups* (Virginia: Al-Anon Family Group Headquarters, 1966), 2. Reprinted by permission of Al-Anon Family Group Headquarters, Inc.
2. Al Mooney, MD, Arlene Eisenberg, Howard Eisenberg, *Recovery* (New York: Workman, 1992), xix.
3. *Al-Anon's Twelve Steps and Twelve Traditions* (Virginia: Al-Anon Family Group Headquarters, 1984), 3. Reprinted by permission of Al-Anon Family Group Headquarters, Inc.
4. *Alcoholics Anonymous: The Story of How Many Thousands of Men and Women Have Recovered from Alcoholism, Third edition* (New York: Alcoholics Anonymous World Services, 1976), 83–84.
5. *One Day at a Time in Al-Anon* (Virginia: Al-Anon Family Group Headquarters, 24th Printing, 1989), 367. Reprinted by permission of Al-Anon Family Group Headquarters, Inc.

Chapter 10: *Providing Natural Consequences*

1. William Glasser, *Reality Therapy* (New York: Harper and Row, 1965), 6.
2. Naomi Glasser, ed., *Control Theory in the Practice of Reality Therapy* (New York: Harper and Row, 1989), xiii.

Chapter 11: *Stories of Empowerment*

1. *Al-Anon's Twelve Steps and Twelve Traditions*, 3. Reprinted by permission of Al-Anon Family Group Headquarters, Inc.
2. *Alcoholics Anonymous: The Story of How Many Thousands of Men and Women Have Recovered From Alcoholism*, 83–84.
3. *Alcoholics Anonymous*, 83–84.

Index

A

abusing, as diagnosis, 78–79

abusiveness, 121, 140

acceptance
> of child's addiction, 188–189
> of power greater/higher than self, 18–19, 162–164, 167–169
> of social use of alcohol, xiii, 8
> of three Cs (cause, control, cure), 180–181

action plans for families
> communicating with school personnel, 21–22
> educating selves about alcoholism/drugs, 22
> finding assessment professionals, 22

addiction vs.dependency, 11–13

adolescence, development during
> defined, 26
> developmental tasks during, 27–30
> experimentation with drugs and alcohol during, 32
> myths of
>> consistent development during, 25
>> homogeneity of teens as group, 24
>> pathological behavior to be expected, 23–24
>> teens as children, 24–25
>> as transitional stage, 25
> normal behavior during, 26–27
> puberty, defined, 26
> reasons for alcohol and drug use during, 31–32

adolescent treatment programs, 240

age of teens
> at first experiment with marijuana, xiv
> when starting to drink alcohol, xiv

aggressiveness, 121, 140

Al-Anon, Families Anonymous
> benefits of, time needed to feel, 21
> contact information for, 21, 248–249
> emotional responses to, 18–21
> higher/greater power, role of concept in, 18–19
> meetings, format of, 18
> no dues or fees for, 19
> not religious fellowships, 18
> overview of, 17–21
> spiritual aspects of, 18–19
> *See also* spirituality; treatment

alcohol, 253

alternatives to traditional recovery programs, 83

amphetamines, 253–254

anger
> leading to communication problems, 140–143
> as normal reaction to situation, 112
> of parents at premature discharge from treatment, 100
> of parents at school professionals, 153–154
> at teens rather than at disease, 72–73

articles, lists of, 240, 241–242

communication patterns
    as family roles, 143–144
    individual roles
        drug/alcohol abuser teenager,
            144–145
        family hero, 144, 147–149,
            151–152
        lost child, 144, 149
        mascot, 144, 149–150
        prosecutor, 144, 146–147
        scapegoat (rebellious child),
            144, 150
        super parent/grandparent,
            144–147
    leading to loneliness and despair,
        138–143
    of parents and families, 139–143
    predictability of, 144
    recognizing need for improvement
        of, 153–154
    of siblings, 147–150
    taken on without knowledge of
        doing so, 144
    See also defenses to pain
confidentiality, 55–56
consequences of alcoholism/addiction.
        See disease, alcoholism
        and addiction as
consequences of behaviors of abusers/
        addicts. *See* natural and
        logical consequences
controlling others, 121, 140
costs of treatment
    financial, 84–86, 92
    vs. possible consequences without
        treatment, 83–84
    See also insurance
counseling, 14
counseling referrals
    contact information for, 249–250
court consequences, as leverage, 60–67
crack, xiv, 256
Crowley, Jim
    behaviors in schools, effect of drugs
        on, 33–34
    denial of problems by community
        members, 48
    suspension from school,
        alternatives to, 65

D

defenses to pain, 112–116, 140–143
    See also communication patterns
delusion. *See* denial and rationalization
denial and rationalization
    of alcoholics and addicts, 14, 55
    of community members, 48
    and distorting the truth, 75–76
    high level of in early recovery,
        159–161
    of parents/family members, 14–15,
        32–33, 80–82, 164
    when seeking mood swing, 9–11
    See also emotional consequences of
        disease for alcoholics/
        addicts; enabling
dependency *vs.* addiction, 11–13
dependent, as diagnosis, 79
dependent or not abusing, as diagnosis,
    77–78
depressants, 253
depression, 13, 58
designer drugs (fentanyl-based), 255
despair and hopelessness, 73, 119,
    142–143, 153
developmental tasks during adolescence
    alcohol and drug use, impact on,
        30–32
    cognitive development, 28–29
    physical development, 27–28
    social and emotional development,
        29–30
diagnosis
    complicating factors in, 75–76
    criteria for found in DSM IV, 74
    options for
        abusing, 78–79
        dependent, 79
        not abusing or dependent,
            77–78
    professionals qualified to give, 74
    See also assessment
*Diagnostic and Statistical Manual of
        Mental Disorders IV* (DSM
        IV), 74
disease, alcoholism and addiction as
    biological nature of, research into, 7
    biopsychosocial model of, 5–7

natural and logical consequences
(*continued*)
    concepts in reality therapy,
        199–200
    court leverage as means of applying,
        208
    definitions of, 201
    earning privileges during recovery,
        211
    facing reality of choices, 210–211
    gifts and changes from
        for addicts/alcoholics, 216–217
        for families, 213–214
        for parents, 214–216
    importance of, 200–202
    learning about, 206–207
    meaning of, for alcoholics/addicts,
        206
    school leverage as means of
        applying, 208
    selecting by parents, 208
    structure important to parents, 213
    vs. punishment, 202–203
    See also letting go
normal, definition of, 26
not abusing or dependent, as diagnosis,
    77–78
notes, 261–263
nutritional needs, neglect of, 11

O

"One Day at a Time," 225–226
opium/opiates/opiate-like drugs, xiv,
    256–257
options for treatment
    clinical care criteria
        abstinence potential, 91
        acceptance/resistance of
            treatment, 91
        acute intoxication/withdrawal
            potential, 90–91
        emotional/behavioral
            conditions/complications,
            91
        family/caregiver functioning,
            91
        physical health conditions/
            complications, 90
        recovery environment, 91

disagreements about placement,
    92–93
    and parents, 92
outcome statistics of treatment
    programs, 85–86

P

pain
    behaviors for dealing with,
        140–143
    defenses to, 112–116
    importance of to continued
        recovery, 169–170
    interference of with recovery,
        119–120
    often unexpressed by parents,
        105–106
    of siblings of drug/alcohol abusers,
        147–150
parents. *See* parents and families
parents and families
    action plans, suggestions for, 21–22
    attempts to rescue abusers by,
        13–14
    benefits of treatment for, 87
    changes in after applying natural/
        logical consequences,
        213–216
    communication patterns of,
        143–153
    confusion about teen behaviors,
        dealing with, 46–49
    dysfunctional families of, 151–153
    emotional burnout of, 140–142,
        179–180
    feelings during assessment process,
        69–73
    helped by drug court involvement,
        65
    letting go by, 178–198
    making changes through treatment,
        96–98
    manipulation of teens by, 131
    marriage of parents, effect of disease
        on, 16–17
    overcompensation by, 16
    parenting traps for, 131–134

parents and families (*continued*)
  progression of effects of disease on, 13–17
    attempting to adjust, 13–15
    becoming isolated, 15–16
    surrendering to the illness, 16–17
  quitting abuse by, not answer for teens, 82
  self-examination of, 116–117
  siblings, family roles of, 147–150
  starting treatment, 94–96
  stress-related illnesses in, 16, 117, 123–125
  taking care of selves
    action plans for, 21–22
    attending individual therapy, 137
    communicating with schools, 21–22
    examining ways of dealing with pain, 116–118
    exercising, 137, 180
    finding adolescent treatment programs, 137
    finding assessment professionals, 22
    finding/attending support meetings, 17–21, 79, 118, 155
    forming partnerships with schools and courts, 217–218
    gaining education and information, 22, 79, 137, 154–155
    meeting other parents, 49
    reading from DSM IV, 79
    seeking therapy for childhood issues, 118
    talking with each other, 154
    during treatment process, 102
    using music/films/books, 118, 136–137, 155
    while working on letting go, 198
    during work on recovery, 176–177
  in treatment, 93–102
PCP (phencyclidine), 257

peer pressure, 3
Positive Choices for Ongoing Recovery, 170–171
power greater/higher than self, 18–19, 162–164, 167–169
powerlessness, 164–167
Prayer, Serenity
  as means of empowerment, 222–224
  text of, 177
  use and practice of, 222–224
premature discharge from treatment, 100–101
pretreatment, 78–79
prevention, contact information for, 250–252
promises
  believing in, 230–238
  inspiration provided by, 177
  as means of empowerment, 231–238
prosecutor, as family role, 144, 146–147
psilocybin (mushrooms), 257
puberty, defined, 26
  See also adolescence, development during
punishment *vs.* natural and logical consequences, 202–203
  See also natural and logical consequences

R

raising responsible children. *See* natural and logical consequences
rationalization. *See* denial and rationalization; enabling
Rational Recovery (RR), 83
raves, xiv
reasons for abuse and dependency
  during adolescence, 31–32
  biopsychosocial disease model, 5–7
  not absolutely known, 5
recordings to explore feelings, list of, 244
recovery
  and Alcoholics Anonymous, 156–158
  definition of, 156

Serenity Prayer
    as means of empowerment,
        222–224
    text of, 177
    use and practice of, 222–224
shame, 71, 112
siblings, communication patterns of,
    147–150
signs and symptoms of abuse. *See*
        warning signs of possible
        abuse
slogans
    daily life, role in, 224–230
    "Easy Does It," 224–225
    "How Important Is It?", 226–227
    "Let Go and Let God," 227–230
    "Live and Let Live," 227
    as means of empowerment,
        224–230
    "One Day at a Time," 225–226
"Special K" (ketamine hydrochloride),
    257
spirituality
    acceptance of power greater than
        self, 18–19, 162–164,
        167–169
    as aspect of Al-Anon, Families
        Anonymous, 18–19
    God, meaning of in Step Three,
        168–169
    not same as religious beliefs or
        practices, 18–19
    See also recovery
sponsors, 169, 171–173
stages in disease
    chronic and fatal addiction, 11–13
    learning about mood-altering
        substances, 8
    moving from harmful abuse to
        dependency, 10–11
    seeking the mood swing, 8–10
starting treatment, 94–96
Steps of recovery
    to improve serenity, 220
    list of, 158, 220
    as means of empowerment,
        219–220
Steps to a Relapse, 138–139
steroids, 258

stimulants, 253–256
stories of empowerment. *See*
        empowerment, stories of
street names of drugs, 253–259
stress
    feelings/actions in response to, 104,
        152
    illnesses from, in families, 16, 117,
        123–125
    relief off as part of letting go,
        179–180
suicide, 12–13, 153
super parent/grandparent, as family role,
    144–147
support groups and meetings
    Adult Children of Alcoholics, 118
    contact information for, 21,
        248–249
    Families Anonymous, Al-Anon,
        Nar-Anon, overview of,
        17–21
    finding by families, 17
    shopping around for and trying out,
        21
    See also Al-Anon, Families
        Anonymous; Nar-Anon
surprise, 71–72
surrender, 159–161, 164–167

T

taking care of selves by parents and
    families
    action plans for, 21–22
    attending individual therapy, 137
    communicating with schools,
        21–22
    examining ways of dealing with
        pain, 116–118
    exercising, 137, 180
    finding adolescent treatment
        programs, 137
    finding assessment professionals, 22
    finding/attending support meetings,
        17–21, 79, 118, 155
    forming partnerships with schools
        and courts, 217–218
    gaining education and information,
        22, 79, 137, 154–155

About the Author

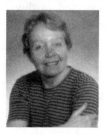

Nikki Babbit, PhD, has spent the past 35 years working with adolescents and families, first as a high school teacher, and then as a school psychologist and adolescent and family therapist working in schools, psychiatric wards, and public health clinics. In 1980, she had the opportunity to be the founding Director of the New Directions Residential and Outpatient Treatment Programs for Drug/Alcohol Dependent Adolescents in Cleveland, Ohio, which literally began in her living room. She retired from her management responsibilities at New Directions fifteen years later, in 1995, to devote time to her writing, but still maintains clinical ties as a consultant, therapist, and facilitator/teacher in a weekly education/support group for parents of adolescent alcoholics/addicts.

Nikki has been a consultant to schools, juvenile justice facilities, and youth agencies across the United States, on youth and family issues and drug/alcohol abuse and dependency issues. In 1989, she traveled to the Soviet Union to help begin AA and Al-Anon, which had been prohibited by the government despite their success in over 120 countries around the world. The following year she was invited to Moscow to speak about western alcoholism treatment methods at the joint Soviet-American Conference on Alcoholism.

Nikki has been married to Harold Babbit since 1965 and they have three children, one of whom is recovering. She was the child and stepchild of alcoholics. She is the author of the booklet *Is My Child Chemically Dependent?* (Community Intervention Press, 1988), and lives in Shaker Heights, Cleveland, Ohio.

Ms. Babbit's photograph is from MotoPhoto.

Colophon

Patient-Centered Guides are about the experience of illness. They contain personal stories as well as a mixture of practical and medical information. The faces on the covers of our Guides reflect the human side of the information we offer.

The cover of *Adolescent Drug and Alcohol Abuse: How to Spot It, Stop It, and Get Help for Your Family* was designed by Kathleen Wilson using Adobe Photoshop 5.0 and QuarkXPress 3.32 with Berkeley fonts from Bitstream. The cover photo is from Picture Quest, and is used with that company's permission. The cover mechanical was prepared by Ellie Volckhausen.

The interior layout for the book was designed by Alicia Cech, based on a series design by Nancy Priest and Edie Freedman. The interior fonts are Berkeley and Franklin Gothic. The text was prepared by Mike Sierra using FrameMaker 5.5.6. Illustrations were created by Rhon Porter and Robert Romano using Adobe Photoshop 5.0 and Macromedia FreeHand 8.0. The text was copyedited by Lunaea Hougland and proofread by Jeff Holcomb. Maureen Dempsey and David Futato provided quality assurance. The index was written by Kate Wilkinson. Interior composition was done by Maeve O'Meara, Sarah Jane Shangraw, and Gabe Weiss.

Patient-Centered Guides™

Questions Answered
Experiences Shared

We are committed to empowering individuals to evolve into informed consumers armed with the latest information and heartfelt support for their journey.

When your life is turned upside down, your need for information is great. You have to make critical medical decisions, often with information that seems little to go on. Plus you have to break the news to family, quiet your own fears, cope with symptoms or treatment side effects, figure out how you're going to pay for things, and sometimes still get to work or get dinner on the table.

Patient-Centered Guides provide authoritative information for intelligent information seekers who want to become advocates for their own health. The books cover the whole impact of illness on your life. In each book, there's a mix of:

- **Medical background for treatment decisions**
  We can give you information that can help you work with your doctor to come to a decision. We start from the viewpoint that modern medicine has much to offer and we discuss complementary treatments. Where there are treatment controversies, we present differing points of view.

- **Practical information**
  Once you've decided what to do about your illness, you still have to deal with treatments and changes to your life. We cover day-to-day practicalities, such as those you'd hear from a good nurse or a knowledgeable support group.

- **Emotional support**
  It's normal to have strong reactions to a condition that threatens your life or that changes how you live. It's normal that the whole family is affected. We cover issues such as the shock of diagnosis, living with uncertainty, and communicating with loved ones.

Each book also contains stories from both patients and doctors—medical "frequent flyers" who share, in their own words, the lessons and strategies they have learned while maneuvering through the often complicated maze of medical information that's available.

We provide information online, including updated listings of the resources that appear in this book. This is freely available for you to print out and copy to share with others, as long as you retain the copyright notice on the printouts.

www.patientcenters.com

Other Books in the Series

Cancer

Advanced Breast Cancer
A Guide to Living with Metastatic Disease, Second Edition
By Musa Mayer
ISBN 1-56592-522-X, Paperback, 6" x 9", 544 pages, $24.95 US, $36.95 CAN

"An excellent book...if knowledge is power, this book will be good medicine."
—*David Spiegel, MD, Stanford University, Author,* Living Beyond Limits

Cancer Clinical Trials
Experimental Treatments and How They Can Help You
By Robert Finn
ISBN 1-56592-566-1, Paperback, 5" x 8", 232 pages, $14.95 US, $21.95 CAN

"I highly recommend this book as a first step in what will be for many a difficult, but crucially important, part of their struggle to beat their cancer."
—*From the* Foreword *by Robert Bazell, Chief Science Correspondent for NBC News Author,* Her-2: The Making of Herceptin, a Revolutionary Treatment for Breast Cancer

Colon & Rectal Cancer
A Comprehensive Guide for Patients & Families
By Lorraine Johnston
ISBN 1-56592-633-1, Paperback, 6" x 9", 556 pages, $24.95 US, $36.95 CAN

"I sure wish [this book] had been available when I was first diagnosed. I wouldn't change a thing: informative, down-to-earth, easily understandable, and very touching."
—*Pati Lanning, colon cancer survivor*

Non-Hodgkin's Lymphomas
Making Sense of Diagnosis, Treatment & Options
By Lorraine Johnston
ISBN 1-56592-444-4, Paperback, 6" x 9", 584 pages, $24.95 US, $36.95 CAN

"When I gave this book to one of our patients, there was an instant, electric connection. A sense of enlightenment came over her while she absorbed the information. It was thrilling to see her so sparked with new energy and focus."
—*Susan Weisberg, LCSW, Clinical Social Worker, Stanford University Medical Center*

Patient-Centered Guides
Published by O'Reilly & Associates, Inc.
Our products are available at a bookstore near you.
For information: **800-998-9938** • **707-829-0515** • **info@oreilly.com**
101 Morris Street • Sebastopol • CA • 95472-9902
www.patientcenters.com

Child/Adolescent Health

Adolescent Drug & Alcohol Abuse
How to Spot It, Stop It, and Get Help for Your Family
By Nikki Babbit
ISBN 1-56592-755-9, Paperback, 6"x 9", 304 pages, $17.95 US, $26.95 CAN

"The clear, concise, and practical information, backed up by personal stories from
people who have been through these problems with their own children or clients,
will have readers keeping this book within easy reach for use on a regular basis."
> —*James F. Crowley, MA President, Community Intervention, Inc.*
> *Author,* Alliance for Change: A Plan for Community Action on Adolescent
> Drug Abuse

Bipolar Disorders
A Guide to Helping Children & Adolescents
By Mitzi Waltz
ISBN 1-56592-656-0, Paperback, 6" x 9", 464 pages, $24.95 US, $36.95 CAN

"As bipolar disorders are becoming more commonly diagnosed in children and adolescents, a readable, informative guide for these youths and their families is certainly
needed. This book certainly fits the bill. It covers all of the major topics that are of
greatest importance to guide parents and families on the topic of pediatric bipolarity."
> —*Robert L. Findling, MD, Director, Division of Child and Adolescent*
> *Psychiatry, Co-director, Stanley Clinical Research Center, Case Western*
> *Reserve/University Hospitals of Cleveland*

Childhood Cancer
A Parent's Guide to Solid Tumor Cancers
By Honna Janes-Hodder & Nancy Keene
ISBN 1-56592 531-9, Paperback, 6"x 9", 544 pages, $24.95 US, $36.95 CAN

"I recommend [this book] most highly for those in need of high-level, helpful
knowledge that will empower and help parents and caregivers to cope."
> —*Mark Greenberg, MD, Professor of Pediatrics, University of Toronto*

Childhood Cancer Survivors
A Practical Guide to Your Future
By Nancy Keene, Wendy Hobbie & Kathy Ruccione
ISBN 1-56592-460-6, Paperback, 6" x 9", 512 pages, $27.95 US, $40.95 CAN

"Every survivor of childhood cancer should read this book."
> —*Debra Friedman, MD, Assistant Professor of Pediatrics, Division of*
> *Hematology/Oncology, Children's Hospital and Regional Medical Center,*
> *Seattle, WA*

Patient-Centered Guides
Published by O'Reilly & Associates, Inc.
Our products are available at a bookstore near you.
For information: **800-998-9938** • 707-829-0515 • info@oreilly.com
101 Morris Street • Sebastopol • CA • 95472-9902
www.patientcenters.com

Child/Adolescent Health

Childhood Leukemia
A Guide for Families, Friends & Caregivers, Second Edition
By Nancy Keene
ISBN 1-56592-632-3, Paperback, 6" x 9", 520 pages, $24.95 US, $36.95 CAN

"What's so compelling about *Childhood Leukemia* is the amount of useful medical information and practical advice it contains. Keene avoids jargon and lays out what's needed to deal with the medical system."
—The Washington Post

Obsessive-Compulsive Disorder
Help for Children and Adolescents
By Mitzi Waltz
ISBN 1-56592-758-3, Paperback, 6" x 9", 408 pages, $24.95 US, $36.95 CAN

"More than a self-help manual…a wonderful resource for patients and professionals alike. Highly recommended."
—*John S. March, MD, MPS, Author,* OCD in Children and Adolescents: A Cognitive-Behavioral Treatment Manual

Pervasive Developmental Disorders
Finding a Diagnosis and Getting Help
By Mitzi Waltz
ISBN 1-56592-530-0, Paperback, 6" x 9", 592 pages, $24.95 US, $36.95 CAN

"Mitzi Waltz's book provides clear, informative, and comprehensive information on every relevant aspect of PDD. Her in-depth discussion will help parents and professionals develop a clear understanding of the issues and, consequently, they will be able to make informed decisions about various interventions. A job well done!"
—*Stephen M. Edelson, PhD, Director, Center for the Study of Autism, Salem, Oregon*

Inspiration/Human Interest

The Nicholas Effect
A Boy's Gift to the World
By Reg Green
ISBN 1-56592-860-1, Paperback, 6" x 9", 272 pages, $19.95 US, $29.95 CAN

"This book is a story of grace, dignity, and how one family turned senseless tragedy into a life-affirming gesture."
—*Robert Kiener,* Reader's Digest

Patient-Centered Guides
Published by O'Reilly & Associates, Inc.
Our products are available at a bookstore near you.
For information: **800-998-9938** • **707-829-0515** • **info@oreilly.com**
101 Morris Street • Sebastopol • CA • 95472-9902
www.patientcenters.com

Neurological

Hydrocephalus
A Guide for Patients, Families & Friends
By Chuck Toporek and Kellie Robinson
ISBN 1-56592-410-X, Paperback, 6" x 9", 384 pages, $19.95 US, $28.95 CAN

"In this book, the authors have provided a wonderful entry into the world of hydrocephalus to begin to remedy the neglect of this important condition. We are immensely grateful to them for their groundbreaking effort."
—Peter M. Black, MD, PhD, Franc D. Ingraham Professor of Neurosurgery, Harvard Medical School, Neurosurgeon-in-Chief, Brigham and Women's Hospital, Children's Hospital, Boston, Massachusetts

Partial Seizure Disorders
Help for Patients and Families
By Mitzi Waltz
ISBN 0-596-50003-3, Paperback, 6" x 9", 325 pages, $19.95 US, $29.95 CAN

"Mitzi Waltz has provided people with epilepsy and their families a compassionate yet supremely practical book. She explains complicated medical information in lucid, detailed language, and provides an excellent guide to navigating the maze of educational and healthcare bureaucracies. *Partial Seizure Disorders* is a book to be referred to often and shared with others."
—Patricia Murphy, Editor, Epilepsy Wellness Newsletter

Disabilities

Choosing a Wheelchair
A Guide for Optimal Independence
By Gary Karp
ISBN 1-56592-411-8, Paperback, 5" x 8", 192 pages, $9.95 US, $14.95 CAN

"I love the idea of putting knowledge often possessed only by professionals into the hands of new consumers. Gary Karp has done it. This book will empower people with disabilities to make informed equipment choices."
—Barry Corbet, Editor, New Mobility Magazine

Patient-Centered Guides
Published by O'Reilly & Associates, Inc.
Our products are available at a bookstore near you.
For information: **800-998-9938** • **707-829-0515** • **info@oreilly.com**
101 Morris Street • Sebastopol • CA • 95472-9902
www.patientcenters.com

Disabilities

Life on Wheels
For the Active Wheelchair User
By Gary Karp
ISBN 1-56592-253-0, Paperback, 6" x 9", 576 pages, $24.95 US, $36.95 CAN

"Gary Karp's *Life on Wheels* is a super book. If you use a wheelchair, you cannot do without it. It is THE wheelchair-user reference book."
— *Hugh Gregory Gallagher, Author, FDR's Splendid Deception*

General Interest

Working with Your Doctor
Getting the Healthcare You Deserve
By Nancy Keene
ISBN 1-56592-273-5, Paperback, 6" x 9", 384 pages, $15.95 US, $22.95 CAN

"*Working with Your Doctor* fills a genuine need for patients and their family members caught up in this new and intimidating age of impersonal, economically driven healthcare delivery."
— *James Dougherty, MD, Professor Emeritus of Surgery, Albany Medical College*

Your Child in the Hospital
A Practical Guide for Parents, Second Edition
By Nancy Keene and Rachel Prentice
ISBN 1-56592-573-4, Paperback, 5" x 8", 176 pages, $11.95 US, $17.95 CAN

"When your child is ill or injured, the hospital setting can be overwhelming. Here is a terrific 'road map' to help keep families 'on track.'"
— *James B. Fahner, MD, Division Chief, Pediatric Hematology/Oncology, DeVos Children's Hospital, Grand Rapids, Michigan*

Making Informed Medical Decisions
Where to Look and How to Use What You Find
By Nancy Oster, Lucy Thomas & Darol Joseff, MD
ISBN 1-56592-459-2, Paperback, 6" x 9", 392 pages, $17.95 US, $26.95 CAN

"I will buy this book for all of our clinic sites and our patient library. It is a terrific reference."
— *Laurie Lyckholm, MD, Medical Oncologist, Massey Cancer Center, Medical College of Virginia*

Patient-Centered Guides
Published by O'Reilly & Associates, Inc.
Our products are available at a bookstore near you.
For information: **800-998-9938** • **707-829-0515** • **info@oreilly.com**
101 Morris Street • Sebastopol • CA • 95472-9902
www.patientcenters.com